JOINT REPLACEMENTS

A Patient's Handbook

✓ **Can we avoid it?**
✓ **Stories of real patients**
✓ **Key to success**

Dr. Narayan Hulse

MS, DNB, MRCS(UK), MCh (Liv), FRCS(Orth)UK
Director of Orthopaedics and Joint Replacement
Surgery.
Fortis Hospital, Bannergatta Road, Bangalore,
560076, India

STARDOM BOOKS

STARDOM BOOKS
WORLDWIDE
www.StardomBooks.com

STARDOM BOOKS

A Division of Stardom Publishing and infoYOGIS
Technologies.
105-501 Silverside Road

Wilmington, DE 19809

FIRST EDITION JANUARY 2021

Stardom Books

Joint Replacement
A Patient's Handbook

Dr. Narayan Hulse

p. 278
cm. 13.5 X 21.5

Category:
Non-Fiction/Medical/Orthopedics

ISBN-13: 978-1-7332116-8-0

BEFORE YOU START...

The aim of the book is to elucidate the general principles of joint replacement surgery. It can neither replace your surgeon nor substitute a surgical discussion with him. A surgeon's training of over a decade, and the cumulative experience he gains from his patients are invaluable.

DEDICATED TO

My teachers from three continents who
have trained me,
My patients, each of whom has taught me
something new,
My friends and colleagues, they're my forever
pillars of support,
My hospital — my temple of worship, and finally,
To the lovely family I am blessed with.

Thank you!

CONTENTS

CASE STUDIES

1
INTRODUCTION

One of the key prerequisites for a successful joint replacement surgery is a well-informed patient. Every time I come across a new patient, I am met with a new question that has never been asked by any of my previous patients, and this, I believe without a shadow of a doubt, has added more value to my experience spanning over two decades as a Joint Replacement Surgeon.

Having witnessed an array of clinical interactions with patients suffering from joint pain, I have many clinical encounters to share, and this book has paved the way for me. I have attempted to consolidate my experiences to help the readers understand, decide, and recover from a joint replacement surgery successfully.

Myths

Several medical myths scream for attention; while some are harmless, many are downright dangerous. This may be due to the lack of public awareness or even the

1

fear associated with surgery. These myths result in many patients undergoing different forms of alternative therapies like Ayurveda, homeopathy, magnetotherapy, electrotherapy, and several other remedies, which are not curative. After going through the ordeal, the sad part is that they end up suffering from more pain, feeling depressed, and finally will be in need of a more complicated corrective operation.

Arthritis has become one of the common problems across the world, affecting people of all age groups. There are more than a hundred types of arthritis, and most of them are not curable through medicines and other therapies. Hence, joint replacement surgery becomes inevitable for patients suffering from end-stage joint diseases, for they deal with severe pain, deformity, and immobility.

That said, those patients who have mild arthritis can be relieved of their discomfort with minimal support. For this, however, patients need effective education and assistance to simplify their treatment plans.

Putting things in perspective, joint replacement surgeries are one of the most common operations performed across the world, and in the last fifty years, the demand for this has gone through the roof. Patients who are otherwise crippled with harrowing pain are now witnessing tremendous improvement in their quality of life.

Future

There is a sharp increase in the number of patients diagnosed with arthritis each year across the world. Arthritis is more common in older people, and the number seems to be growing exponentially. In fact, a study by the Centers for Disease Control (CDC) for the National Arthritis Data Workgroup (NADW) had revealed that by 2030, the number of people with arthritis or any other rheumatologic condition would increase by a whopping 44% a surge to 67 million!

In this book on "Joint Replacements - A Patient's Handbook," I have answered over a hundred commonly asked questions by my patients. My belief in educating the population on preventive strategies, the merits of several methods of treatments, and their complications has indeed come true with this book. It is a collection of vignettes from my two decades of clinical experience, and I hope that with this book, I will be able to help you with most of your concerns, if not all, regarding joint replacements. I wish you a happy reading.

Dr. Narayan Hulse

DR. NARAYAN HULSE

4

2
UNDERSTANDING A JOINT

Summary:
Joints where two bones come in contact to provide mobility, have a soft lining called cartilage. This structure is damaged progressively in all types of arthritis. Unfortunately, cartilages have no intrinsic healing capacity, and there are no effective medicines to regenerate them.

Joints are the locations within our body where two or more bones meet. Most of the joints provide a variable amount of mobility to allow a certain degree of movement, as required to function effectively.

Bones provide stability and a framework like a scaffolding for other organs of the body. For example, our shoulder joint has more mobility as it enables us to perform finer activities; however, they are not very stable; they easily dislocate. On the other hand, although our knee joint has only unidirectional movement, they are strong, and they rarely dislocate. Knee joints have to be strong as they have to carry our body weight.

Structure of a Joint

As I mentioned earlier, a typical joint involves two bones meeting each other (figure 1). The presence of cartilage, a resilient, smooth elastic rubber-like tissue, protects the bone's end surface in the joint and prevents them from rubbing against each other. Put simply, it acts as a cushion and reduces the friction between the bones. The cartilage is progressively damaged in all types of arthritis, resulting in increased friction and pain.

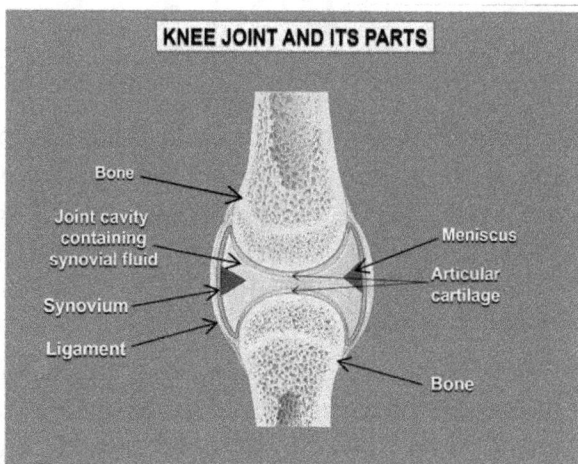

Figure 1: Knee joint and its parts

Synovium is a soft-membrane that lines the joint from the inside, and its outer surface adheres to the joint capsule. Cells in the synovium produce synovial fluid, which lubricates the joint. When the cartilage gets damaged, the synovial fluid production increases up to three times. This excessive synovial fluid can distend the joint and can cause further pain. This fluid can be removed easily for testing in laboratories to make the diagnosis of Arthritis.

Another vital aspect of joints is the ligaments - the tough, sturdy rope-like structures that connect the bones and hold them from abnormal movements. Ligaments most commonly get ruptured in sports injuries causing instability or buckling of the knee joint.

On the other hand, the meniscus is a cushion-like structure in the knee joints that are made of tough cartilage materials. However, the menisci can get torn during sports and other similar activities.

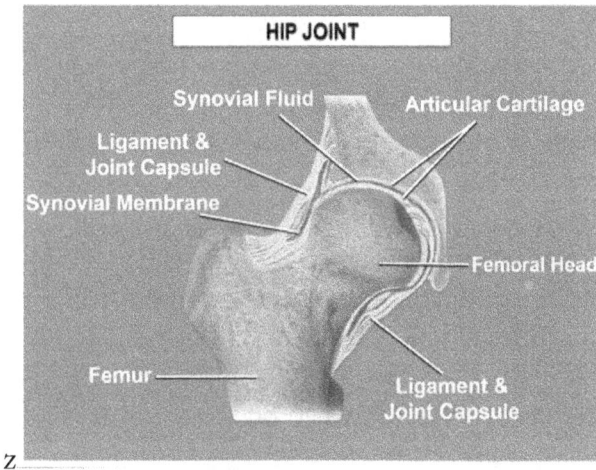

Figure 2: Hip joint and its parts

Types of Human Joints

1. Ball-and-Socket Joints:

Ball-and-socket joints consist of a cup-like socket and a ball-like head that rotate inside the socket [figure 2]. They allow us to move backward, forward, sideways, and make rotatory movements. Hip and shoulder joints are typical examples. These joints allow a more massive range of actions than other joints and hence are more prone to dislocations.

2. Hinge Joints:

These are common synovial joints present in ankles, elbows, and knee joints [Figure 1]. Also present in fingers, and toes, hinge joints allow bending and straightening movements while also helping us in activities that involve excessive pressure on bones.

3. Pivot Joints:

These joints allow limited rotating movements, just like the neck's cervical spine.

4. Ellipsoidal Joints:

These joints allow all types of movements except pivotal movements.

5. Fixed Joints:

As the name suggests, these joints are fixed and have minimal movement. Skull, joints between the vertebrae, and the joint between the tooth and the jaw are some places where fixed joints can be seen.

Importance of Cartilage in Joints

Cartilage cells, also called chondrocytes, are sparsely distributed in a medium called the extracellular matrix. The extracellular matrix mainly consists of water, collagen, and proteoglycans, with other non-collagenous proteins and glycoproteins.

These constituents of the matrix help retain water, which is crucial for the cartilage's unique mechanical properties.

Articular cartilage or joint cartilage is a highly specialized connective tissue of about two to four millimetres thick. It provides a smooth and lubricated surface for the joint by facilitating the transmission of loads with less friction. For context, the cartilage is also called 'Hyaline cartilage'; 'Hyali' means glass in Greek. Adding on, the cartilage is devoid of blood vessels, lymphatics, nerves and is subject to a harsh biomechanical environment.

Cartilage Damage in Arthritis

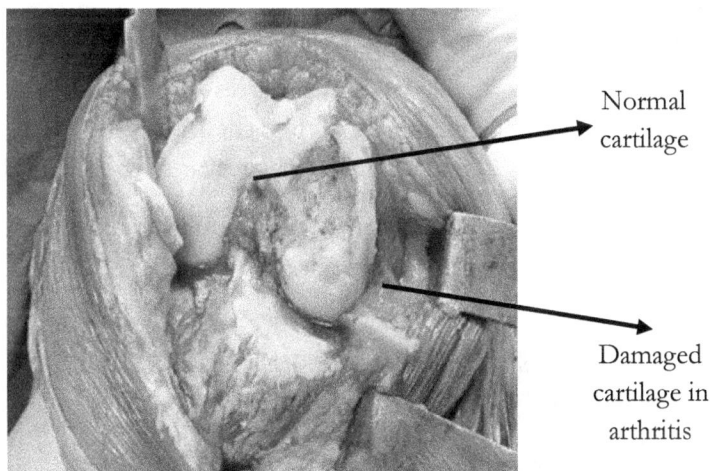

Normal cartilage

Damaged cartilage in arthritis

Figure 3: Inside of an arthritic joint, as seen during a knee replacement

Despite its unique structure, flexibility, and strength, cartilage can get damaged in conditions such as trauma, accidents, and age-related wear and tear. Various arthritic conditions like osteoarthritis, rheumatoid arthritis, ankylosing spondylitis can also lead to the weakening or wear and tear of the cartilage.

Depending on the amount of cartilage loss, bones

might even start rubbing against each other, causing pain, restriction in movements, and difficulty in walking. The complex structure of articular cartilage also makes the treatment of the cartilage-wear challenging. The absence of blood vessels, nerves, and lymphatics is the reason for articular cartilage's limited capacity for intrinsic healing and repair.

When the joint cartilage has thinned out, the body may produce a limited amount of poor-quality cartilage or bone, leading to irregular, bumpy outgrowths called osteophytes. This process results in an uneven joint surface, causing an impediment to the movements. These damages are usually progressive and are not reversible.

Therefore, following a healthy lifestyle, maintaining ideal body weight, managing the fractures around the joint promptly, and treating conditions like rheumatoid arthritis early on becomes crucial. All of these points mentioned above are discussed in detail in the following chapters.

References:

1) Vaienti E, Scita G, Ceccarelli F, Pogliacomi F. Understanding the human knee and its relationship to total knee replacement. Acta Biomed. 2017 Jun 7;88(2S):6-16.

2) Bullough P: The pathology of osteoarthritis. In Osteoarthritis. Goldberg V, Mankin H. Philadelphia: WB Saunders, 1992:39–69.

3) L J Sandell, T Aigner: Articular cartilage and changes in arthritis. An introduction: cell biology of osteoarthritis. Arthritis Res. 2001;3(2):107-13.

4) Alice J Sophia Fox, Asheesh Bedi, Scott A Rodeo: The basic science of articular cartilage: tructure, composition, and function.: Sports Health. 200 9 Nov;1(6):461-8.

3
ARTHRITIS AND CAUSES OF JOINT PAIN

Summary:
Joint pain can be a result of any disorder associated with the joints. Osteoarthritis, also called 'wear and tear,' is the most common cause of joint pain in the elderly, followed by rheumatoid arthritis.

Joint pain is a prevalent problem among adults, and arthritis is a significant contributor to joint pains in those aged 18 and above. A study conducted by the National Arthritis Data Workgroup in 2019 had revealed that more than 22% of American adults [over 52.5 million people] had arthritis and that by 2030, the number of people with arthritis would rise to 67 million.

The number of people affected by arthritis is increasing at an alarming rate in India as well. As per data collected in 2017, over 180 million people in India had arthritis. This prevalence is higher than diabetes, AIDS, and even cancer. Every year, around 14% of the Indians seek doctor's help for their joint-related problems.

Causes of Joint Pain

Joint pain is a broad, non-specific terminology. Any disturbances in the joints' complex mechanisms can cause pain. However, chronic conditions like arthritis are more concerning. Aging is one of the main factors that contribute to joint pain.

Fractures and injuries are treated differently depending on their severity. If the joint mechanism is not restored after sustaining a fracture, patients will eventually develop a painful degeneration of the involved joint.

Infections are caused by the invasion of a plethora of microorganisms, which can cause further damage in the joints, and if this is not treated on time, it could lead to permanent joint damage.

What is Arthritis?

The word 'arthritis' includes a group of painful conditions characterized by the destruction of joint cartilage. Arthritis is derived from the Greek word 'arthro,' meaning joint, and 'itis'- meaning inflammation.

There are over one hundred conditions which can be grouped under the term arthritis. The common types of arthritis are:

1. Osteoarthritis
2. Rheumatoid arthritis
3. Gouty arthritis
4. Ankylosing spondylitis
5. Psoriatic arthritis
6. Post-traumatic arthritis
7. Septic arthritis
8. Reactive arthritis

9. Hemochromatosis
10. Ochronotic arthritis

Osteoarthritis [OA]

Osteoarthritis is the most common form of arthritis and is seen in the elderly, commonly women. This disease evolves with age and is commonly termed as 'wear and tear of aging.' OA leads to joint cartilage getting worn out progressively, resulting in painful movements.

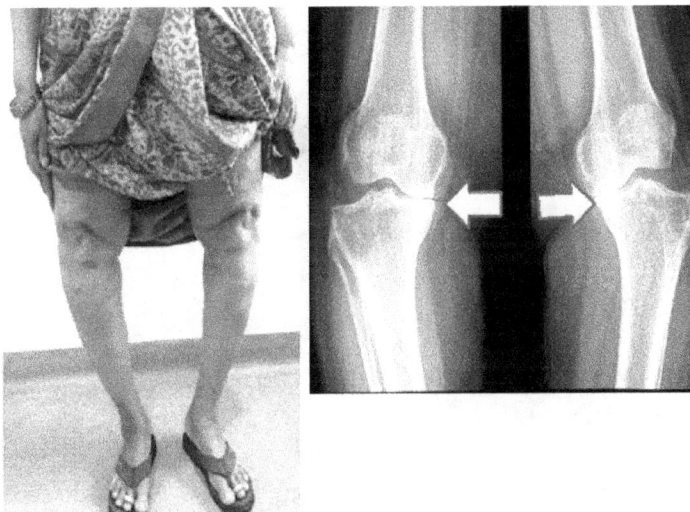

Figure 4: Varus deformity due to loss of cartilage on the inner side of the knees

Two out of three obese people will develop symptomatic knee osteoarthritis at least once in their lifetime. Nearly 50% of the people are prone to develop symptomatic knee osteoarthritis by the age of 85.

Doctors are seeing an increasing number of people with this condition lately. OA mainly affects the knee joint, followed by the hip, spine, wrist, and hand. In rare cases, even other joints can be affected. The process of 'wear and tear' leads to the thinning of the cartilage until it is completely depleted.

This wear occurs asymmetrically, resulting in a thinner cushion of cartilage in some places and thicker cartilage in the others. A bow leg deformity occurs commonly because of the severe thinning of the cartilage on the knee's inner side (figure 4).

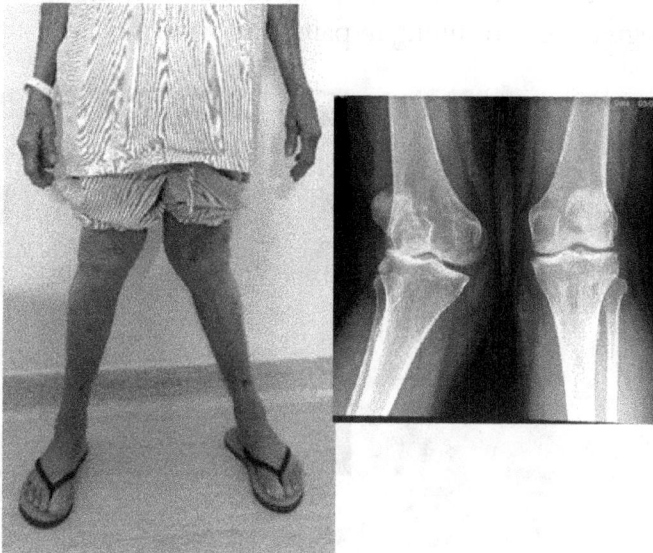

Figure 5: Valgus deformity due to loss of cartilage on the outer side

People can also rarely develop a 'knock-knee' or a 'valgus deformity' when the knee's outer side is more worn-out than the inner side (figure 5). Some people with arthritis cannot straighten their knees fully; this disabling deformity is called 'flexion deformity.'

Rheumatoid Arthritis [RA]

Rheumatoid arthritis is the second most common form of arthritis, after osteoarthritis. It can affect people of a much younger age group. A form of this condition called 'Juvenile Rheumatoid Arthritis' affects young children. RA also occurs more frequently if you have a family history, and relatively, women are more prone to this disease than men.

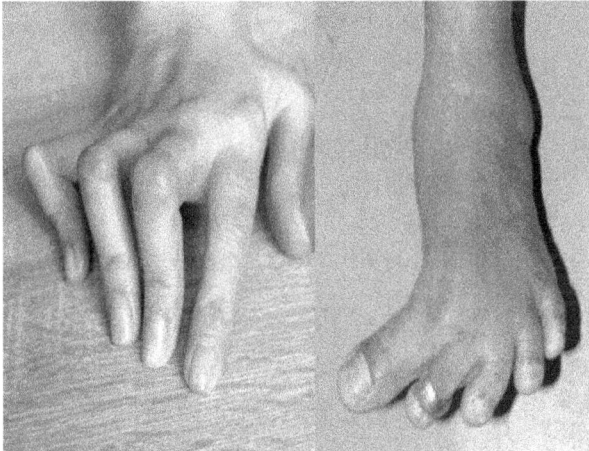

Figure 6: Rheumatoid hand and foot

RA is an autoimmune condition wherein our immune mechanism damages the body cells resulting in joint pains. This disease eventually takes over the entire body, including the heart, lungs, wrists, hands, and knees, causing severe disability.

Hence, this condition should be diagnosed early and treated with medications to prevent its progression and complications. There is no single test that will diagnose RA. However, your doctor will diagnose the condition by looking at the following factors:

1. Morning stiffness lasting more than thirty minutes.
2. Symmetrical involvement of small joints of the hand and feet.
3. Multiple joints' swelling for more than six weeks.
4. Appearance of skin nodules called Rheumatoid nodules.
5. Positive Rheumatoid Factor in blood test (RF).
6. Positive anti-CCP in the blood test.
7. Increased inflammatory markers in the blood tests like ESR and CRP.

Other Common Types of Arthritis

Gouty Arthritis:
It is a condition due to decreased body's ability to degrade uric acid, a protein metabolism product. Crystals of uric acid are deposited in the joints, especially in the big toe, causing severe pain. Gouty arthritis is usually treated with medications and diet.

Ankylosing Spondylitis:
It is a genetic disease that causes a severe form of arthritis at a very young age. Commonly found in men, patients develop severe stiffness in the spine and hip joints in this condition. Hip replacement surgery could be the only solution to improve their mobility.

Psoriatic Arthritis:
This is a common form of skin disease that affects the knee joints, hips, and fingers. However, joint replacements are required in rare cases only. There is also a higher risk of artificial joint infections in psoriasis.

Post Traumatic Arthritis:

A variety of fractures and other trauma can damage the joints and cartilage that may progress to become secondary osteoarthritis. This condition will require treatments similar to osteoarthritis.

Septic Arthritis:

Infection in the joints can cause severe destruction of the cartilage. This condition is considered an orthopaedic emergency, and in this case, patients may require emergency surgery.

If the treatment gets delayed, the joints might not return to its normal condition and might eventually need a joint replacement.

References:

1) Pujalte GG, Albano-Aluquin SA: Differential Diagnosis of Polyarticular Arthritis. Am Fam Physician. 2015 Jul 1;92(1):35-41.
2) Mandl LA: Osteoarthritis year in review 2018: Clinical. Osteoarthritis Cartilage. 2019 Mar; 27(3):359-364.
3) Smolen JS, Aletaha D, McInnes IB: Rheumatoid arthritis. Lancet. 2016 Oct 22;388(10055):2023-2038.

4
WHAT IS A JOINT REPLACEMENT?

Summary:
Joint replacement is a surgical procedure in which parts of an arthritic or damaged joint are removed and replaced with painless artificial materials such as metals. Joint replacements are one of the most successful and popular surgical operations.

Joint replacement, also known as Arthroplasty, is an orthopaedic surgical procedure where damaged joint surfaces are replaced with an artificial material called 'prosthesis.' This procedure enables the patient to move their joints freely without experiencing any pain.

Total knee replacement is the most commonly performed procedure, followed by total hip replacement surgery. Replacements of the entire shoulder, elbow, ankle, wrist, and small joints in the hands and fingers are also performed based on different conditions. However, they are not as common as knee and hip replacements.

History of Development of Total Hip Arthroplasty

Hip replacement is termed as "the operation of the 20th century" — thanks to the exceptional improvements seen in the quality of life post-operation. Various types of hip surgeries have been performed over the last three hundred years, and this evolution from basic surgeries to the most advanced total hip replacements is commendable. The goal of relieving pain and restoring mobility has been successfully achieved.

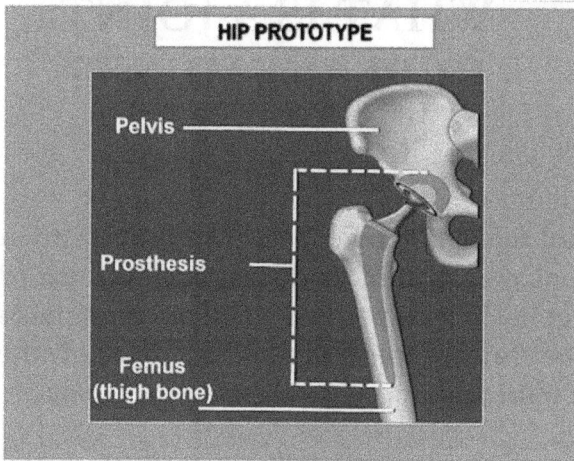

Figure 7: Hip prototype

In 1891, Professor Themistocles Glück, from Germany, made the first attempt to replace the ball of the hip joint. He used an ivory ball to replace the damaged joint in a tubercular patient and presented his research at the 10th International Medical Conference in Berlin in 1890. In 1925, an American surgeon, Smith Petersen (1886- 1953), provided synthetic inter-positional Arthroplasty with a mould prosthesis using glass. Unfortunately, this practice led to the moulds being broken, yielding poor results, and Petersen ended up abandoning it permanently. He then tried again with materials like celluloid, Bakelite, and Pyrex, and in 1937, his dentist suggested he tried Vitallium. For context, Vitallium is a cobalt-chromium-molybdenum alloy with higher resistance to fatigue or fracture than either stainless steel or titanium.

After an extensive study, in the same year, Smith Petersen released Vitallium joints. He later went on to develop over 500 Vitallium moulds that proved to show encouraging results.

In 1940, Austin Moore, an American orthopaedic surgeon, a pioneer in the use of the femoral-head prosthesis and Vitallium, introduced the first metal prosthesis at John Hopkins Hospital. The procedure replaced the proximal twelve inches of the femur with a custom-made Vitallium prosthesis. Moore, along with Harold Ray Bohlman, refined their implant and, in 1952, described a model that featured a fenestrated stem to allow bone ingrowth. Both the designs were produced in collaboration with Howmedica Inc. (at the time, Austen Laboratories, now merged with Stryker® Corporation, East Rutherford, New Jersey, United States). Later, these became the first hip arthroplasty products to be widely distributed.

The first to use a metal-on-metal prosthesis regularly was an English surgeon, George McKee. In 1953, he began to use the modified Thompson stem (a cemented hemiarthroplasty used for neck of femur fracture treatment) with a new one-piece cobalt-chrome socket as the new acetabulum. This prosthesis had a reasonable survival rate, about 74%. Yet this method grew unpopular by the mid-1970s due to the local effects of metal particles seen during revision surgery for prosthetic failure.

An eminent orthopaedic surgeon Sir John Charnley, who worked at the Manchester Royal Infirmary and Wrightington Hospital in the UK, is considered the father of the modern hip replacement surgery. Hip implants that he designed in the early 1960s are identical in principle to the prostheses used today. Charnley's design consisted of three parts - a metal femoral stem, a polyethylene acetabular component, and acrylic bone cement. It was referred to as the low friction arthroplasty as Charnley advocated the use of a small femoral head, which reduced 'wear' due to its smaller surface area.

Later in the 1970s and 1980s, the uncemented type of total hip replacement became popular in parts of North America. Cementless components used biological fixation to ensure the implant holds to the patient's bone. This was achieved by generating compression using a slightly larger implant than the size of the bone-bed; the cementless implants thus got the name 'press-fit' devices. Furthermore, hybrid devices combine different components; they are either a cemented stem with an uncemented cup or a cemented cup with an uncemented stem. The latter implant type is referred to as a reverse hybrid.

Over the next three decades, metal-on-metal, resurfacing designs, ceramic articulations were developed, and there was also further development in cross-linking the polyethylene material to decrease the wear.

History of Development of Total Knee Arthroplasty

Modern total knee replacement has evolved continuously over the years and is one of the most critical medical interventions of the 20th century. Scientists have tried their hands at several techniques to relieve people of their joint pains. In 1860, Stanislas Verneuil, a French physician, and surgeon suggested the interposition of soft tissues like muscle, and subsequently, pig bladder, nylon, facia, and cellophane were used. However, most of them failed very early due to infection and other mechanical failures.

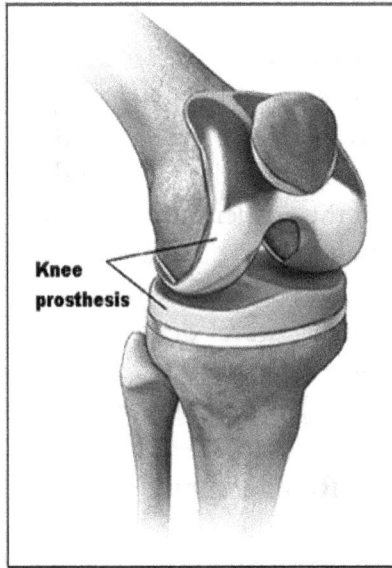

Figure 8: Prototype of a total knee replacement

In 1951, Waldius, a Swedish Orthopaedic surgery educator, introduced a hinged joint made of acrylic, which was later replaced by metal in 1958. Unfortunately, this hinged joint suffered from an early failure. In the 1950s, Duncan C. McKeever introduced the theory of unicompartmentalized replacement for only one compartment of the knee joint. McKeever asserted that replacement of the entire knee was unnecessary if only one knee compartment was affected. At the same time, McKeever also introduced metallic tibial components that resurfaced only the tibial plateau.

In the 1960s, Sir John Charnley developed hip prosthesis using metal and polyethylene surfaces. This, in turn, prompted similar developments in knee replacements. Gunston, a Canadian surgeon, came up with a partial knee replacement in 1968 with a cobalt-chromium alloy and high-density polyethylene for the first time, similar to the materials used today.

During the 1970s, the femoral and tibial joint surfaces were completely replaced by metal and polyethylene called the 'total condylar knee'; this formed the basis for the most modern designs. In the 1970s and 1980s, metallurgy, the geometry of the artificial joint, and fixation techniques improved tremendously. Further refinement in the sizing of the components and the option of replacing the kneecap or patella were developed. In the last two decades, computer navigation and robotic-assisted total knee replacements have revolutionized the space.

Future of Joint Replacement

There has been a significant rise in the number of people undergoing joint replacement surgeries in recent times. This growing awareness and increasing acceptance of the procedure could be due to multiple reasons. However, the rising number of elderly patients diagnosed with arthritic conditions, obesity, and other lifestyle disorders seem to top the list.

It is speculated that the number of joints implanted will increase by 174% in the United States by 2030, and the number of surgeries performed across the globe will see a two-fold increase in the next two decades. This rise will be much higher in developing economies like India because of the increasing awareness and growing number of older people.

References:

1) Narayan Hulse: Total knee replacement in arthritis - Current Concepts. Chapter 9. Frontiers in Arthritis, Ashish Anand (Ed). 2017, Vol 1, 105-127.

2) Learmonth ID, Young C, Rorabeck C: The operation of the century: total hip replacement. Lancet.2007 Oct 27;370(9597):1508-19.

3) Carr AJ, Robertsson O, Graves S, Price AJ, Arden NK, Judge A, Beard DJ: Knee replacement. Lancet. 2012 Apr 7;379(9823):1331-40.

4) Stephen Richard Knight, Randeep Aujla, Satya Prasad Biswas: Total Hip Arthroplasty – over 100 years of operative history. Orthopedic Reviews 2011; volume 3:e16.

5) Pablo F Gomez, Jose A Morcuende: Early attempts at hip arthroplasty--1700s to 1950s. Iowa Orthop J, 2005;25:25-9 health. 2009 Nov;1(6):461.

Case 1: Victim of Alternative Therapy

Mrs. Rani (name changed), a 55-year-old widow of a bank manager, had been suffering from severe rheumatoid arthritis. After pulling through ten years of continuous rheumatological treatments, her rheumatologist finally suggested her to undergo knee replacements.

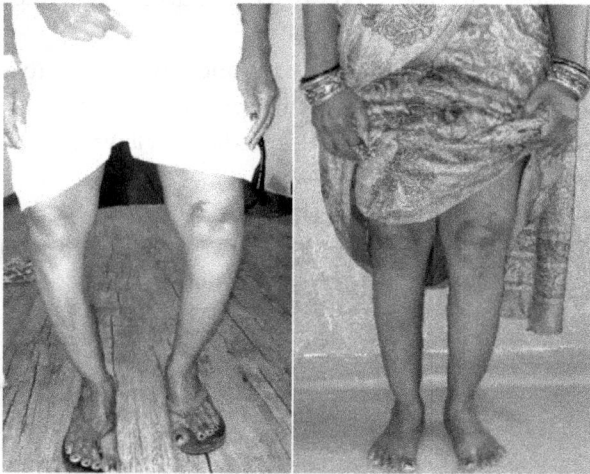

**Figure 9: [Left]Bent knee before surgery
[Right] Straight legs after surgery**

Mrs. Rani had been delaying her knee replacements for two reasons. Firstly, since she lives all by herself, there was no one to take care of her post-operation. Secondly, her financial status made it difficult for her to afford the surgery as her husband's pension was her sole income.

It was during this time that she learned about the Ayurvedic therapy 'Panchakarma.' Traditional practitioners commonly use this treatment, irrespective of the disease's stage, diagnosis, or efficacy. Unfortunately, none of these therapies can actually cure rheumatoid arthritis. Mrs. Rani underwent the treatment for a few weeks but found no relief. Nothing met her expectations, and she ended up spending a lot of money (Rs 3,000 per session). This is the reason why it is crucial to administer only scientific and proven therapy. Otherwise, people might end up losing time, money, health, and even confidence.

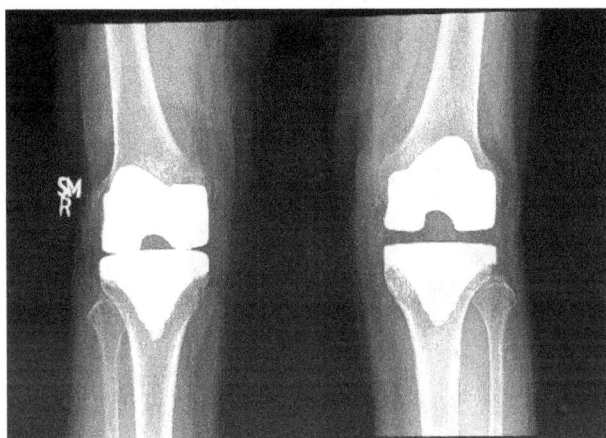

Figure 10: Both knee joints with knee replacement components

Finally, after a year, I conducted both knee replacements simultaneously on her. She had already developed a lot of deformities, osteoporosis, and clinical depression. Rehabilitation took a long time, but Mrs. Rani did exceptionally well. She was fully mobile in about three months after the surgery.

Case 2: Husband Carried Her in His Arms for Five Years!

Imagine a 40-year-old lady being dependent on someone to even go to the washroom. Her husband had to literally carry her from room to room (figure 11). However, because of his daily job at a manufacturing company, the husband had no option but to leave her alone most of the days. With two small children at home, she could not even visit her parents as they lived far away.

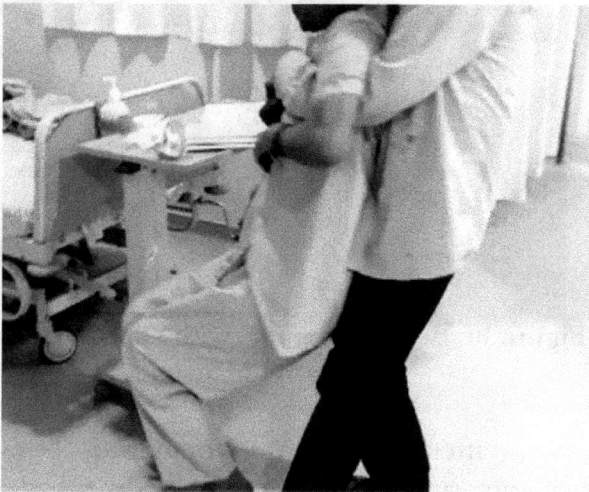

Figure 11: Husband carrying her to all basic daily activities

The lady had chronic rheumatoid arthritis. The disease was so aggressive that it could not be controlled even after administering several medications. Gradually, she developed severe swelling, pain, and stiffness in both her knees; they started bending, and she found it difficult to even straighten the knee. Her knees were stuck in a folded position [about 100 degrees (figure 12)], and she experienced similar issues in other joints as well.

Although I had advised her to undergo both knee replacements long ago, she ended up delaying it for more than six months because of social and financial constraints.

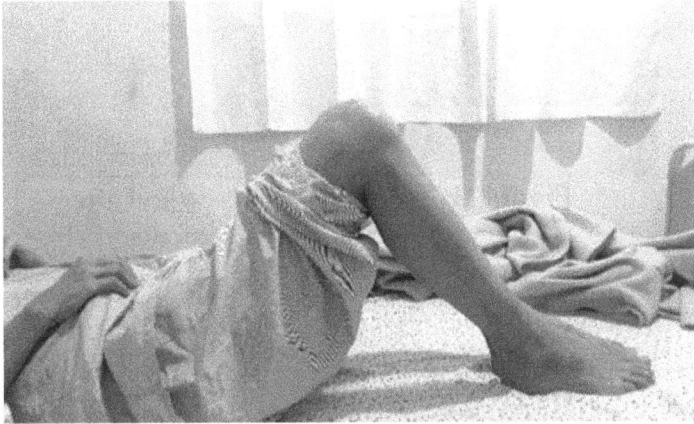

Figure 12: Both knees are bent and locked at 100 degrees

Having tried several unsuccessful medications and alternative therapies, she was also not sure about the surgery outcomes. She had almost given up. However, in the end, I conducted both knee replacements sequentially at an interval of five days. Correcting such severe deformity is exceedingly difficult, but with the help of computer navigation, we achieved complete correction.

Astonishingly, she recovered quite quickly and was discharged in just ten days. She continued her exercises for a long time and is now completely independent. After a while, she got back to me all excited and told me that nobody could even make out that she had undergone a knee operation.

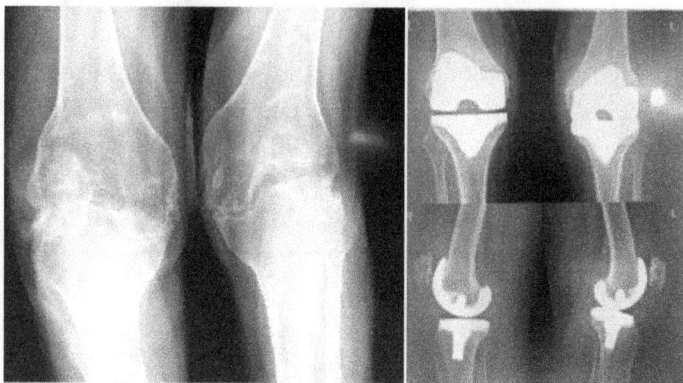

Figure 13: X-rays taken before and after both total knee replacements

Case 3: TKR For Both Husband and Wife

Mrs. Parimala (name changed), a retired teacher, had been suffering from severe knee pain for many years because of osteoarthritis. After several months of non-operative treatment, she underwent both knee replacements, showed speedy recovery, and returned to her daily activities.

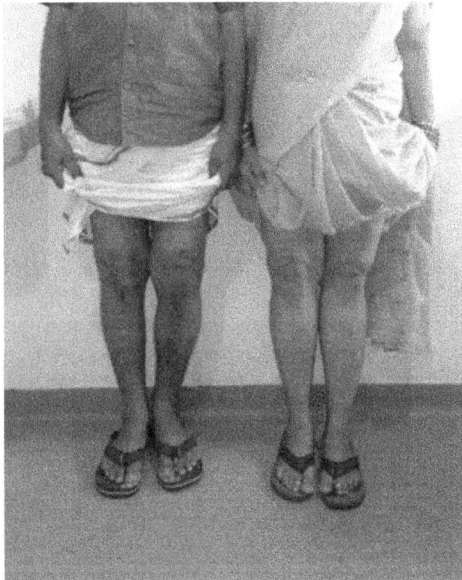

Figure 14: Both knee replacements seen in the husband-wife duo

Mrs. Parimala's husband, also a victim of osteoarthritis was inspired by how his wife's knee replacements had improved her quality of life. Three years after his wife's surgery, he also underwent both knee replacements. As expected, he was delighted with the outcome. These instances stand proof to the fact that knee replacements are indeed a reliable option.

Case 4: Sixteen Knee Replacements in the Same Family!

This is a story of the members of an extended family and their relatives, all sharing the same surname. This particular case study demonstrates the high success rates of knee replacements. Every person who underwent this surgery recommended it to another, and this way, I have performed a total of sixteen knee replacements from this family in the past seven years.

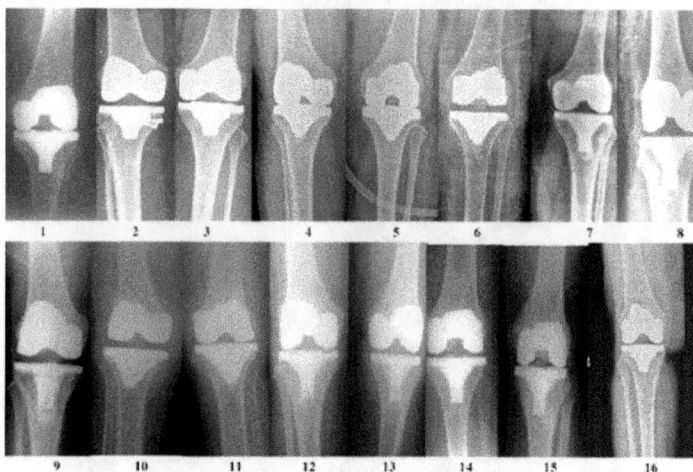

Figure 15: X-ray of the sixteen knee replacements

The first patient was a 60-year-old lady who had suffered from severe right knee pain; it took quite a lot of time for her to consider a knee replacement. She was convinced to undergo a knee replacement only after a doctor in her own family reassured her and accompanied her to the hospital for consultation. She eventually came around. We operated on her right knee in 2011. As her quality of life improved tremendously post-surgery, the news spread like wildfire. In a couple of years that followed, I performed 14 more knee replacements from this family. The 16th knee replacement in this series was the first patient herself who returned for her second knee replacement. This was also conducted very successfully, making TKR surgery 100% successful in the entire family.

5
HOW TO AVOID A JOINT REPLACEMENT?

Summary:
It is important to take preventive methods to avoid a surgery. If you look after your knees from a young age, you may be able to save your knees.

Orthopaedic surgeons often face these questions.

- 'Is it possible to regenerate damaged cartilage with present generation treatments?'
- 'Is there something to prevent it?'
- 'If diagnosed at an early stage, can total knee replacement be prevented?'
- 'Is it possible to regenerate damaged cartilage with any form of surgeries available today?'

It is essential to reiterate the fact that cartilage wear and arthritis are not reversible. People should not try unproven and useless therapies that are commonly advertised and marketed for commercial gain. Talk to your orthopaedic surgeon or rheumatologist about your condition before you undergo any treatment.

The Importance of Weight Loss

Maintaining a healthy weight is crucial for your overall wellbeing as it reduces the risk of heart disease, diabetes, cancer and also eases the pain of arthritis and helps your medicines work efficiently. Obesity is one of the major contributors to joint pain. Every kilogram you gain increases the pressure on your knee; the tension is heightened when you walk, climb, and rise from a sitting posture.

During these activities, the force or pressure on each knee, per step, is equivalent to approximately two to three times a person's total body weight. This is called 'joint reaction force' and is similar to the force generated in a lever mechanism described in physics textbooks.

Therefore, gaining a 15 kilograms of body weight could add up to 45 kilograms of force on each knee, per step. Assuming the average person takes roughly around 2,000 steps per day, this additional force could equal up to 100 extra tons of force on each knee per day. Thus, 15 kilograms of weight loss can dramatically reduce the amount of force on our knees.

Many opt for bariatric surgeries to lose weight. Several studies have also been conducted on the effect of bariatric surgeries on knee pain. Edward et al. had studied 24 patients between 30 and 67 years of age who had lost about 25 kilograms, and it was found that these patients had shown significant improvements in knee stiffness and pain management within six months.

The 'Framingham Osteoarthritis Study' had also shown that if you reduce your body weight by two or three body mass indices, then the risk of developing osteoarthritis would also reduce by 50%. However, the main concern is achieving weight loss. Most of the patients suffering from knee pain and obesity find it very difficult to reduce weight because of their inability to walk and perform other physical activities. Such patients can opt for swimming, low-calorie food, and weight reduction surgeries.

Importance of Aerobic Exercise

Many patients tend to put off their visits to a doctor concerning their knee and hip osteoarthritis with an assumption that joint replacement surgeries would most probably be their final resort. Here is what you need to know. Exercise and weight loss could work like a charm. They could help reduce your knee pain and even prevent the surgery altogether.

Exercises increase your muscular strength, improve the biomechanics of the joint, and help in achieving weight loss. A piece of advice — it is always a good idea to consult a physiotherapist before taking to any exercise. Understanding the proper techniques of various activities is necessary.

According to Brosseau's research study, aerobic exercises contribute to better long-term function in active patients with primary knee osteoarthritis. Home exercise programs and supervised exercise classes can substantially decrease pain and improve body function in patients with knee osteoarthritis.

However, the main problem with these exercise regimens is continuing the exercises at home to a longer duration. If discontinued, all the benefits will be lost within six months.

Listed below are some of the recommended exercises that have been proven useful for knee osteoarthritis:

- Aquatic exercise
- Yoga
- Stretching program
- Quadriceps muscle strengthening
- Range of movement exercises
- Cycling
- Walking

Occupational Hazards

Work-life balance is the buzz word these days. Millennials are struggling to strike a balance between professional and private life. It is important to note that certain occupations can increase the risk of developing osteoarthritis in old age. If you are someone who's also suffering from obesity, it's high time you make necessary lifestyle changes.

There are not many studies and research reports published on this topic, as subjects like these require years of follow-up before reaching any conclusion. However, if you have a job or if you're looking for a job that involves the below-mentioned activities, you must check for a family history of arthritic conditions before committing to the task.

- Kneeling
- Excessive stair climbing
- Jumping
- Vibrating machine tools
- Heavy lifting

Additionally, people who work in the below-mentioned occupations are at higher risk of developing osteoarthritis in old age.

- Floor layers
- Carpenters
- Construction workers
- Agriculture
- Mining
- Plumbers

Many occupations and practices that require extreme and prolonged hours of knee bending, kneeling, squatting, stair climbing, heavy lifting ($\geq$ 10 kg), and jumping have shown to be riskier. Furthermore, standing for long hours ($\geq$ 2 hours per day), and walking more than 3 kilometres per day have also been proven to be an additional issue.

One research by Jakowlev et al. looked into the effect of the aforementioned activities among workers. It was concluded that there was more than a fivefold increase of osteoarthritis in these people after the age of 55 years. Consequently, in another study conducted by Holmberg et al., men who worked in the construction industry for more than 30 years were at 3.7 times greater risk of suffering from OA.

Occupations involving a considerable amount of time in knee straining positions (e.g., floor layers, carpenters, and compositors) were shown to pose higher risks of knee osteoarthritis — especially in those workers aged above 50 years. Workers involved in several other occupations such as construction, firefighting, agriculture, fisheries, forestry, and mining are at an increased risk for knee osteoarthritis.

Among Danish adults, the male floor and bricklayers had an increased risk of developing knee osteoarthritis compared to those who worked in an office environment; the rate depends on the number of years spent in that particular occupation.

Among male healthcare assistants, an elevated risk of developing knee osteoarthritis was seen in those who had worked for more than ten years. An increased risk of developing knee osteoarthritis was also seen in female healthcare assistants and construction workers who had worked for more than five years.

Among male workers employed in the Swedish construction industry, there was a significantly increased risk of surgically treated osteoarthritis in the knee among floor layers, asphalt workers, sheet-metal workers, rock workers, plumbers, bricklayers, wood-workers and concrete workers.

Joint Trauma and Fractures:

As we have discussed in the earlier chapters, cartilage will not regenerate once damaged. If a fracture is passing through the joint invariably, it will damage the cartilage. Surgery is the only option in restoring the normal anatomy of these bones.

If the fracture has healed in an inappropriate position of more than 2 millimetres from its original configuration, then there is a higher risk of developing early osteoarthritis.

An estimated 23% to 44% of intra-articular fractures of the knee will lead to post-traumatic osteoarthritis. Acute mechanical damage from an injury and chronic abnormal joint loading due to change in the weight-bearing axis after trauma, both contribute to cartilage breakdown after an intra-articular fracture.

Ligaments:

Knee ligaments are essential for the stability of the knee. The meniscus is necessary for the normal functioning of the knee. Injuries to these structures will alter the biomechanics around the affected joint, which may contribute to cartilage degradation.

Post-traumatic osteoarthritis arises after joint injury and repetitive and collective trauma associated with recurrent instability; it primarily affects the knee and ankle joints. About 10% of osteoarthritis of the knees and about 78% of the ankle arthritis are due to previous trauma. In the literature, these incidences are not better even after the reconstruction of the ligaments of the knee by surgery.

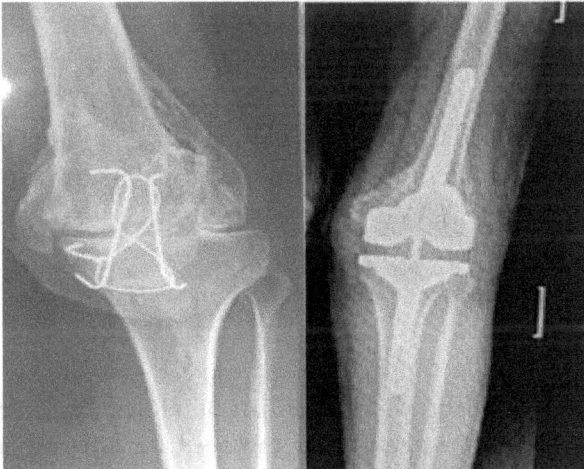

**Figure 16: [Left] Knee fracture with wire fixation
[Right] Needed a knee replacement**

Treating Joint Diseases

Several joint diseases can damage the cartilage eventually. Hence, it is of paramount importance to treat them early and effectively. If a person has rheumatoid arthritis, he or she should be on active treatment at least to considerably delay replacement of the knee or the hip.

Septic arthritis is an emergency condition that usually occurs in children. It should be treated immediately to prevent cartilage damage.

Additionally, steroids can lead to a condition called avascular necrosis (AVN) that can damage the hip joints, and hence this drug should be avoided as much as possible.

Early Corrective Surgeries:

Some corrective surgeries are available for young people to prevent or delay osteoarthritis. For example, someone with a bow leg or a knock-knee from childhood may benefit from surgical correction. Someone with early osteoarthritis may benefit from surgeries like high-tibial osteotomy (HTO), which will be described in detail in the next chapter. People who are developing hip pain after a steroid intake (AVN) may benefit from surgeries like 'Core Decompression'.

References

1) Lajja Rishi, Mohit Bhandari, and Ravindra Kumar; Can bariatric surgery delay the need for knee replacement in morbidly obese osteoarthritis patients. J Minim Access Surg. 2018 Jan-Mar; 14(1): 13–17.
2) Michael DeRogatis, Hiba K Anis, Nipun Sodhi et al: Non- operative treatment options for knee osteoarthritis. Ann Transl Med, 2019 Oct;7(Suppl 7): S245.
3) Christopher Edwards, Ann Rogers, Scott Lynch,et al: The effects of bariatric surgery weight loss on knee

pain in patients with osteoarthritis of the knee. 2012;2012:504189.

4) D.F. McWilliams y, B.F. Leeb z, S.G. Muthuri y: Occupational risk factors for osteoarthritis of the knee: a meta-analysis, Osteoarthritis Cartilage. 2011 Jul;19(7):829- 39.

5) Berran Yucesoya, Luenda E. Charlesb, Brent Bakera, and Cecil M. Burchfiel; Occupational and genetic risk factors for osteoarthritis: A review: Work. 2015 January 1; 50(2): 261– 273.

6) Abbey C. Thomas, Tricia Hubbard-Turner, Erik A. Wikstrom: Epidemiology of Posttraumatic Osteoarthritis. Journal of Athletic Training 2017;52(6):491–496.

7) Sacks JJ, Helmick CG, Langmaid G. Deaths from arthritis and other rheumatic conditions, United States, 1979–1998. The Journal of rheumatology. Sep; 2004 31(9):1823–8.

8) Murphy L, Helmick CG. The impact of osteoarthritis in the United States: A population-health perspective. The American journal of nursing. Mar; 2012 112(3 Suppl 1):S13–9.

9) Sandmark H, Hogstedt C, Vingard E. Primary osteoarthrosis of the knee in men and women as a result of lifelong physical load from work. Scandinavian journal of work, environment and health. Feb; 2000 26(1):20–5.

10) Muraki S, Akune T, Oka H, Mabuchi A, En-Yo Y, Yoshida M, et al. Association of occupational activity with radiographic knee osteoarthritis and lumbar spondylosis in elderly patients of population-based cohorts: A large-scale population-based study. Arthritis Rheum. Jun 15; 2009 61(6):779–86.

11) Holmberg S, Thelin A, Thelin N. Is there an increased risk of knee osteoarthritis among farmers? Apopulation- based case-control study. Int Arch Occup Environ Health.2004 Jun;77(5):345-50.

Case 5: She Flew from Tanzania to India to Correct Her Knock Knees.

Mrs. Ralph (name changed), a 64-year-old lady, had rheumatoid arthritis and was suffering from severe pain and knock-knee. Her legs had bowed out because of arthritis.

Upon recommendation from one of her friends, she traveled from the faraway African country of Tanzania to India to get the surgery done. After a complete assessment of her general health, she underwent both knee replacements simultaneously and it was a success. We performed the surgery using a computer navigation technique.

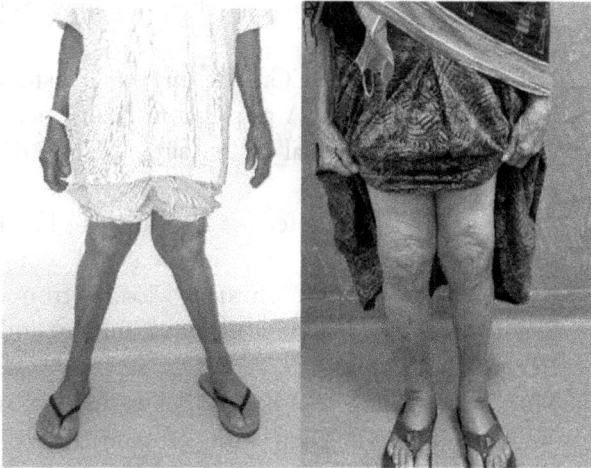

Figure 17: Knock knee before and straight legs after surgery

Mrs. Ralph was pleased to see her both legs straightened after the operation (figure 18). She recovered quite quickly and flew back to her country happily after four weeks.

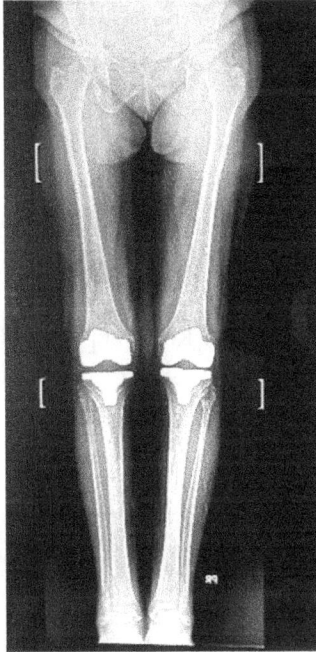

Figure 18: Straight legs after knee replacement surgery

Case 6: Is a Bariatric Surgery Needed to Reduce Weight Before a Knee Replacement?

Mrs Maria (name changed), had been suffering from severe knee pain for several years. With a height of 5 feet 2 inches and a weight of 140 kilograms, obesity was clearly her biggest enemy.

Surprisingly, unlike many others, Mrs Maria was convinced to undergo a knee replacement; however, she had a choice to make. She could either get her knee replaced first and then undergo bariatric surgery to reduce her weight or do the vice versa.

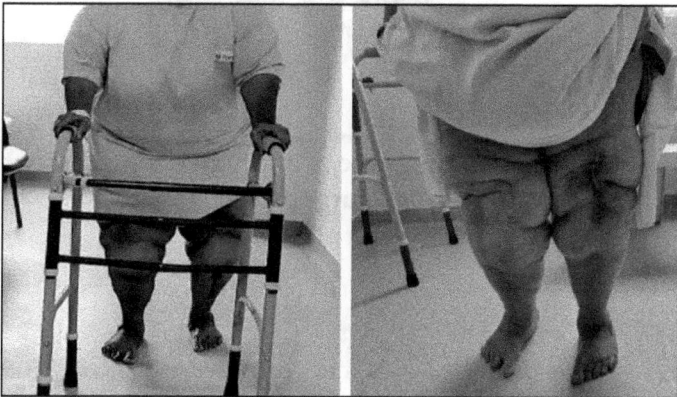

**Figure 19: [Left] Before left knee replacement
[Right] After left knee replacement**

Mrs Maria discussed her situation with several medical experts, including her son, an anaesthetist in the UK. Finally, giving in to her frustration of increasing body weight, she underwent bariatric surgery five years ago.

Although the surgery was a success, Mrs Maria was not entirely benefited. She failed to follow the exercise regimen owing to her knee pain. The pain in both her knees escalated over time, and she could hardly perform any of the house chores; she could not even make slight movements inside the house.

When Mrs Maria approached me, after another five years, she was still weighing about 115 kilograms. X-rays revealed severe wear and tear of the knees, calling for immediate knee replacements. Considering her body weight and other medical conditions, she was a high-risk candidate for knee replacement surgery. However, after all the medical assessments, she finally underwent her left knee replacement.

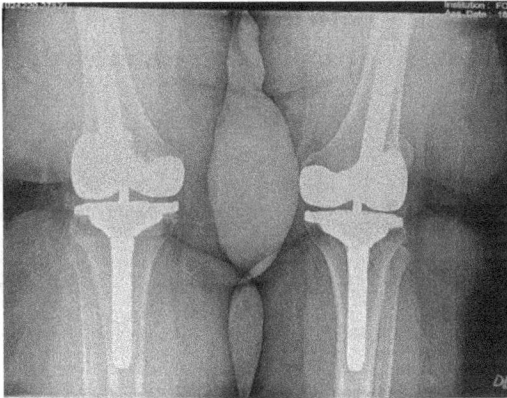

Figure 20: After both knee replacement

Against all the odds, she recovered very quickly and started moving around. Because of obesity and soft osteoporotic bones, we had to use a knee replacement stabilized by stems, (figure 20) which are usually employed during revision knee replacements.

In about four months, she returned happily to have the other knee replaced. Luckily, the second surgery was also a success. Maria recovered quickly and is doing extremely well. However, only time can tell if she will be able to reduce her weight and make the best out of these surgeries.

Case 7: This 90-Year-Old Man Wanted a Knee Replacement.

Mr. Chopra (name changed) is a 90-year-old retired commander from the Indian Airforce. The phrase 'age is just a number' is true in his case. He is always active, cheerful and never misses his daily walks. He also performs simple exercises every day.

As Mr. Chopra recalls, he had suffered an injury on his left knee several years ago, following which he had undergone several courses of physiotherapy, medications to manage the pain. He even had braces on his legs. Despite all this, the pain had progressively worsened over time.

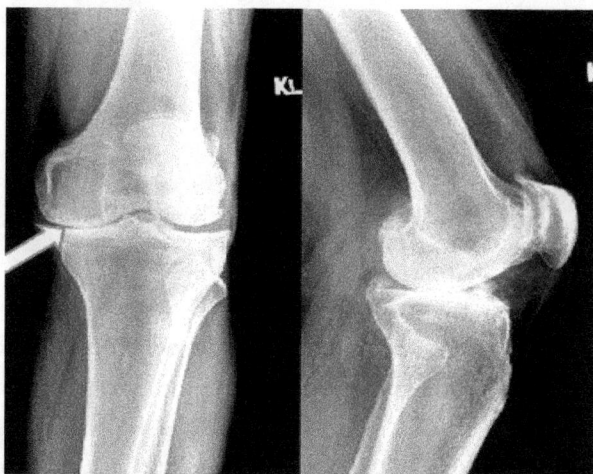

Figure 21: Radiograph showing two bones of the knee rubbing at each other

When I saw him, he was limping and suffering from quite a lot of knee pain. He was extremely healthy otherwise, both physically and mentally. He was a perfect candidate for a knee replacement, unlike other patients of his age.

However, the surgery was a difficult decision to make for both the family and the patient, considering his age. We did our bit by counseling him, along with his family. All the non-operative options available were offered to him. We also explained to him about the risks and benefits of the surgery. Finally, when everybody was in a real dilemma, Mr Chopra took an affirmative decision to undergo the surgery.

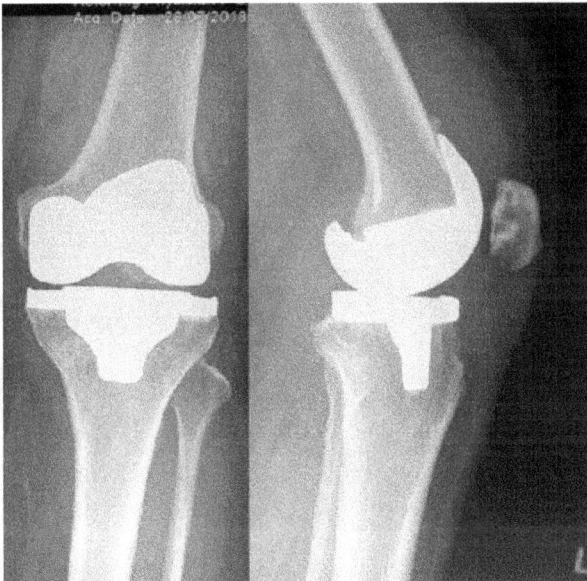

Figure 22: Radiograph after knee replacement

After every possible support and medical care, his operation was conducted successfully (figure 22) He recovered soon and got back to his earlier life within no time.

Case 8: She Was Crippled After a Fracture in Her Knee.

Mrs. Rose (name changed), a 60-year-old lady, had sustained a fracture in her left leg due to a bad fall 12 months ago. She had undergone non-operative treatment in a local hospital [plaster, medicines, and rest]. However, this past year, the pain put her in a lot of misery, and she could hardly use her left leg. She had been walking with the help of a walker with extreme difficulty.

When I saw her, she was in severe pain, and her knee was bent and locked at 20 degrees (flexion deformity). As per the X-ray report, the fracture was partially healed, but not as expected (figure 23). It was healed like a lump of disorganized bone and not like the original bone.

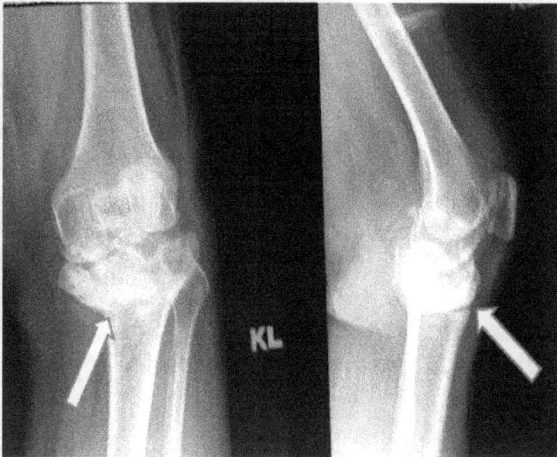

Figure 23: Fracture in the upper part of the leg bone

Fractures involving the joint must be treated with the utmost care and usually with an operation. All the bad fractures involving the knee joints are treated with surgery to bring the broken pieces to their original configuration and are fixed using plates and screws. This will allow stable fixation and also enable early mobilization. If the fractures involving the joints are not appropriately treated, it might lead to stiffness, pain, and even loss of mobility. These joints will degenerate rapidly and may require knee replacements at a very young age itself. Finally, she underwent the knee replacement, and it was one complex operation. As her bone was not healed properly, there was no stable bony base for the knee implant to sit and her bone was very soft (osteoporotic) as she had not walked at all the previous year. Hence, a knee implant with an additional stem was used to provide stability, and supplemental screws were inserted to fix the fracture (figure 24).

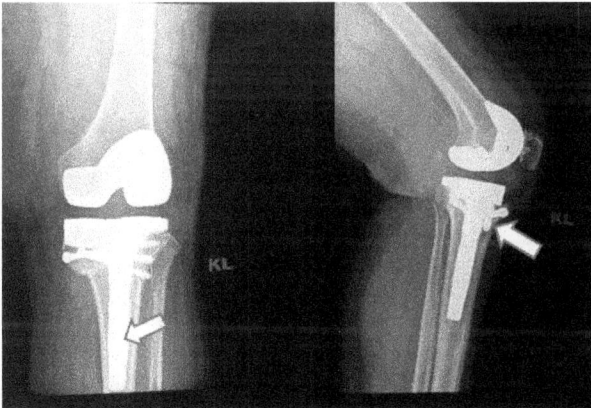

Figure 24: Stem and screws are used along with knee replacements

She had a slow recovery. At about six months post-surgery, she was able to bend her knee at around 100 degrees; other patients usually achieve about 120 degrees by this time. However, her happiness knew no bounds as she was able to walk independently after almost an entire year.

6
ALTERNATIVES TO JOINT REPLACEMENT

Summary:
Even though arthritic cartilages cannot be regenerated, several options are available to relieve pain. These are useful in the early stages of arthritis, young patients or those patients who cannot have a joint replacement surgery.

Arthritis is a common cause of knee pain. Millions of adults who complain of severe joint pains also experience stiffness, decreased movement, which ultimately affects the overall quality of their lives. This condition eventually leads to knee replacement surgery.

It's always better to consider knee replacement surgery as a last resort. There are plenty of other alternatives that you and your surgeon can try out before committing to permanent knee surgery.

I say this because most patients suffer from only mild knee diseases and might not need joint replacement surgery. All they need is some support in their daily activities besides therapies and medications to relieve pain.

Many options are available with a variable amount of safety and efficacy. However, for many treatment modalities, a consensus has not been reached yet, concerning their effectiveness. Therefore, it becomes especially important to understand the risks and benefits of the available options before such treatments are instituted. American Association of Orthopedic Surgeons [AAOS] advises on the management of many such diseases. Some of the recommendations are listed below:

1. Weight loss
2. Aerobic exercises and yoga
3. Heel wedges and braces
4. Acetaminophen and NSAIDs
5. Steroid injections
6. Hyaluronic acid
7. Glucosamine
8. Chondroitin sulphate.

- **Weight loss:** Discussed in chapter 5 (Page 36)
- **Aerobic exercises:** Discussed in chapter 5 (Page 37)

Braces and wedges:

Many types of braces and knee supports are available. Some of them may simply support the knee, while some may offload the knee joint. Some of them are poorly designed and offer no real benefit at all. Hence, they can be very cumbersome to use on a daily basis.

Simple knee-caps made of elastic fabrics may just help to support the knee. Available in different sizes and shapes, there isn't much of a difference between them.

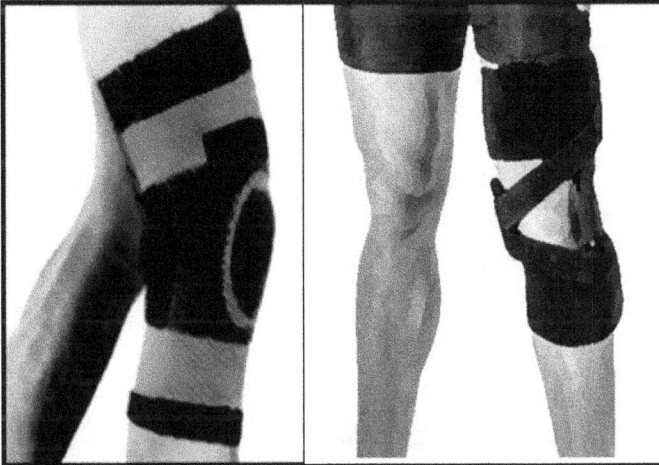

Figure 25: Simple kneecap(left) and knee brace with a hinge(right)

These knee-caps should not be too tight and should not be worn continuously, else they might create passive swelling of the legs and feet.

Braces consist of solid bars on the sides and hinges to allow smooth movements. It looks promising as they might help to offload some weight from thigh to legs bypassing the knee joint, thereby reducing pain.

However, its high cost and the inconvenience experienced while wearing them are the major roadblocks for increased adoption.

A custom-made small wedge can also be inserted inside your shoes (figure 26). This will correct weight-bearing axis of the knee to reduce the lateral thrust. These wedges may be helpful if you have pain only on the knee's inner side.

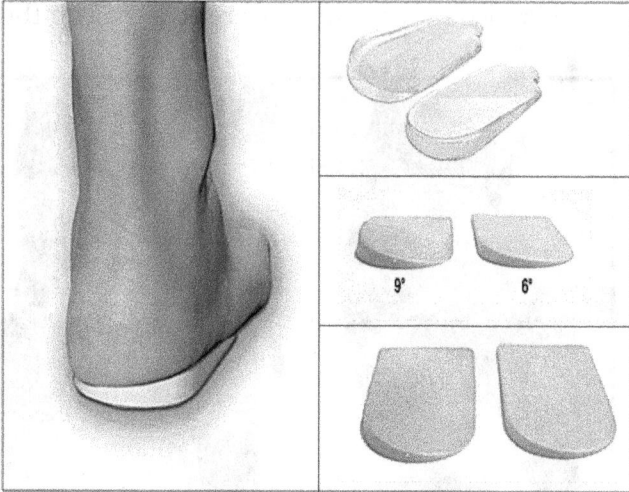

Figure 26: Heel wedges

Non-Steroidal Anti-Inflammatory Agents (NSAIDS)

Pain killers like Paracetamol or Acetaminophen are by far the safest pain-relieving medicines available; they can be administered alone or used in combination with other pain killers (NSAIDS).

However, it can't just be all good things, right? There is an ongoing controversy over the efficacy of NSAIDs as they cause gastritis, gastric ulcers, and bleeding, that might sometimes need intensive care and hospitalization.

Additionally, they cannot be used safely in the presence of renal impairment, diabetes, hypertension, and asthma in elderly patients. However, there are several thousands of people taking these pain killers every day without experiencing any major side effects. If judiciously used, these pain killers can help many people with arthritis and joint pain.

Corticosteroid Injection

Steroids are among the most potent anti-inflammatory agents in the body that reduce the inflammation associated with arthritis and pain. Unlike oral steroids, injections given directly to the joints have very few side effects. Although temporary, this treatment can help those who do not need surgery and also postpone the joint replacements in those who do require surgery.

Triamcinolone, Methyl Prednisolone, Betamethasone are a few among the several types of steroids available in the form of injections. Although they contain the same properties, they vary in terms of efficacy and duration of the action.

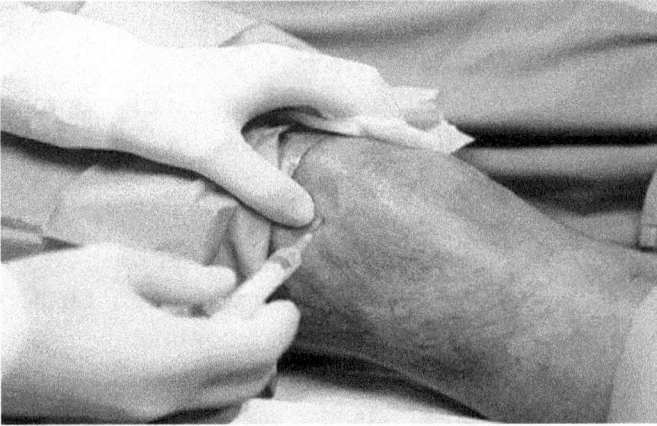

Figure 27: Knee injection being administered Visco-Supplementation

While the injections to knee, ankle, and shoulders are given in out-patient wards, injections to the hip and spine are administered in operation theatres as they need live X-rays. This is done with all sterile precautions taken, and the procedure is carried out under a small dose of local anaesthesia. Patients may resume duties immediately, although they might experience pain the following 24-48 hours; this can be controlled with simple pain killers.

The common problem associated with these injections is the recurrence of pain after a few weeks to a few months. Infection and mild whitish discolouration of the skin are very uncommon. In fact, many orthopaedic surgeons avoid these injections six months to 12 months before a proposed joint replacement surgery because of a slightly higher risk of infections.

This procedure involves the injection of viscous fluid to the knee joints to increase lubrication and ease the pain. Hyaluronic acid is the composition of these injections with variable molecular weights and quantities. These injections provide a combination of viscoelastic properties with associated anti-inflammatory, anabolic, and chondroprotective effects.

However, their efficacy and duration of pain relief are controversial. Generally, they work longer than steroid injections, but the result might vary if the patient is obese and has advanced arthritis. They are usually safe with very few side effects, such as allergies and infections.

Although the American Association of Orthopedic Surgeons is unable to make a recommendation for or against the use of hyaluronic acid injections, in general, the literature supports the use and efficacy of hyaluronic acid.

With the proper patient selection and injection technique, these injections are a viable treatment option for patients with early symptomatic knee osteoarthritis.

Chondro-Protectives or Nutraceuticals

Glucosamine, Chondroitin sulphate, Hyaluronic acid, and Diacerein are widely used to treat early osteoarthritis. Albeit the mode of action and efficacy of these agents are controversial, they continue to be sold as over-the-counter supplements. This has, in fact, increased the sale of these agents without much evidence behind them.

Further research also needs to be performed to define the real potential of these agents to prevent disease progression with well-designed, high-quality, clinical trials. In the absence of definitive regeneration of the arthritic cartilage and long-term beneficial effects, one might question whether these treatments would be reasonable.

Based on the clinical practice guidelines set by the American Association of Orthopedic Surgeons, these supplements are usually not recommended for the management of osteoarthritis.

Platelet Rich Plasma (PRP) Injections

Platelets in our blood contain large amounts of certain biochemical factors necessary for tissue growth and regeneration. A small amount of blood can be removed from your own body and that can be used to extract platelet rich plasma in a simple process. This product is injected into your osteoarthritic knee. There is some scientific evidence to suggest that this injection may repair your worn-out cartilage to some extent and also reduce pain.

However, there is no good evidence yet to suggest this treatment to patients. Its safety, and effectiveness are not yet proven, and the studies are showing conflicting results. American College of Rheumatology and the Arthritis

Foundation (ACR/AF) strongly recommend avoiding this treatment because it has not yet been fully developed and standardized.

Stem Cell Treatment

A stem cell is an immature body cell which can potentially grow to become various mature body cells, depending on the various biological signal and stimulus. Many studies, including animal studies, have shown stem cell treatment to be effective in heart diseases, parkinsonism, muscular dystrophy and other degenerative conditions. The stem cell treatments work by triggering damaged tissues in the body to repair themselves. This is often referred to as "regenerative" therapy.

These stem cells can be grown outside our body using a small amount of blood or other body tissues. However, current evidence is limited to advise this treatment to the public. Food & Drug Administration (FDA) considers stem cell treatment "investigational."

The American College of Rheumatology and the Arthritis Foundation (ACR/AF) do not currently recommend stem cell treatment for OA of the knee. There is no standard procedure for preparing the injection, and there is not enough evidence to prove that it works or is safe.

Operative Treatment

Arthroscopy

This is a keyhole, day procedure that is less popular now because it has minimal or no effect on the real cause of pain in the arthritic joints. Arthroscopic debridement for primary osteoarthritis is controversial.

Some patients may have some relief after arthroscopic knee debridement. Even though 44% of patients have significant decrease in functional pain, 15% of these patients see deterioration within one year. Hence, knee arthroscopy is advocated if the patient has mechanical symptoms (locking and a catch) because of loose, unstable meniscal tears. The other two options, partial knee replacements and high tibial osteotomy, are described in the next chapter.

References

1. DeRogatis M, Anis HK, Sodhi N, Ehiorobo JO, Chughtai M, Bhave A, Mont MA. Non-operative treatment options for knee osteoarthritis. Ann Transl Med 2019;7(Suppl 7):S245.
2. Lucie Brosseau, Lucie Pelland, et al(2004) Efficacy of Aerobic Exercises For Osteoarthritis (part II): A Meta-analysis, Physical Therapy Reviews, 9:3, 125-145.
3. Ferreira RM, Duarte JA, Gonçalves RS : Non-pharmacological and non-surgical interventions to manage patients with knee osteoarthritis: An umbrella review. Acta Reumatol Port. 2018 Jul-Sep;43(3):182-200.
4. Pavelka K, Bruyère O, Cooper C, et al: Diacerein: Benefits, Risks and Place in the Management of Osteoarthritis. An Opinion- Based Report from the ESCEO. Drugs Aging. 2016 Feb;33(2): 75-85.
5. Richmond J, Hunter D, Irrgang. American Academy of Orthopaedic Surgeons clinical practice guideline on the treatment of osteoarthritis (OA) of the knee. J Bone Joint Surg Am 2010; 92:990–993.

Case 9: She Fractured her Leg While Waiting for Knee Replacement

Leela (name changed), a 68- year-old lady was a victim of severe osteoarthritis for six long years (figure 28). The knee pain interfered in all her daily activities, and she was in bad shape. Several modalities of treatments were employed, but nothing really proved successful. Left with no other option, she finally agreed for her left knee replacement.

One morning, just two days before her surgery, she was rushed into the emergency room as she had suffered a fall at home. She had sustained a fracture of the leg-bone just below the knee joint (figure 29). This fall made the situation a little tricky as the doctors had to deal with both fracture and arthritis in the knee.

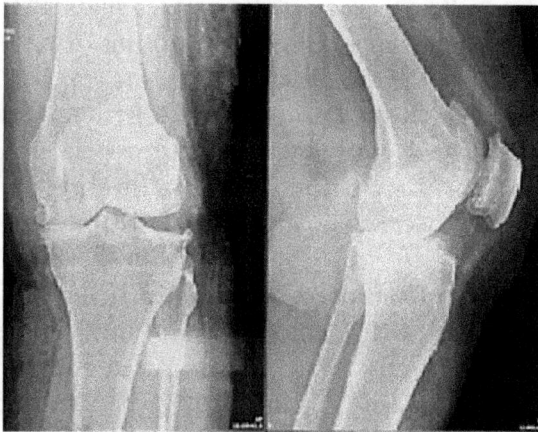

Figure 28: Arthritic knee awaiting a joint replacement

Several patients who struggle to walk because of osteoarthritis in their knees are more susceptible to falls. They should be cautious and stay clear of falls and injuries.

There were two options — one was to treat the fracture first and perform the knee replacement after a gap of three to four months. The second option was to fix both the problems together, which would be a slightly longer operation with associated higher rates of complications. Leela chose the second option. A knee implant with an additional stem was used to fix the fracture simultaneously (figure 30). The fracture healed in three months and she recovered well.

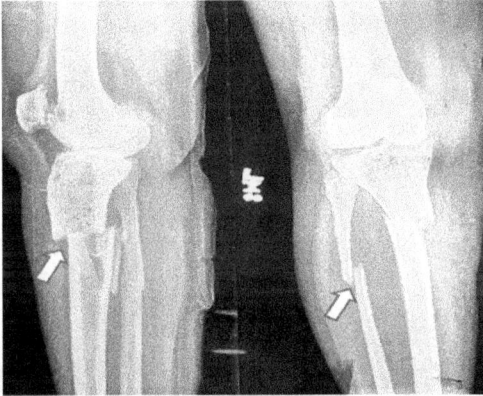

Figure 29: Fracture on the upper part of the leg bone

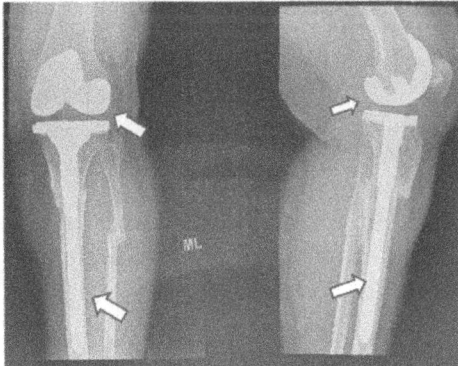

Figure 30: A rod attached to the knee replacement is used to fix the fracture

Case 10: Severe Bow-Legs - Became the 'Talk of the Park'

This 68-year-old lady was suffering from severe knee pain in both her knees due to osteoarthritis. The bowing of her legs made her limp and waddle whenever she walked, and additionally, her bones were weak and worn out severely (figure 31). TKR was the only option that could save her from further misery.

Despite having a loving family capable of taking good care of her, the lady never really considered knee replacement as a viable option. However, her decision changed when her son introduced her to one of his acquaintances, who was leading an active life post-knee replacement surgery.

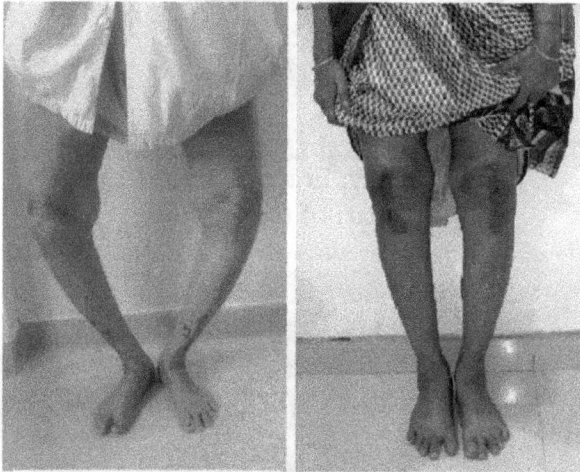

Figure 31: Severe bowing of the legs before surgery and a normally aligned knee after surgery

The implants were fixed firmly inside her weak bones using stems, and to everyone's surprise, she showed rapid recovery. She resumed all her daily activities within three months. She even got back to her evening walks in the park. Looking at her straight knees (figure 33) and completely normal walking style, four of her 'park-friends' with similar conditions also got their knees replaced!

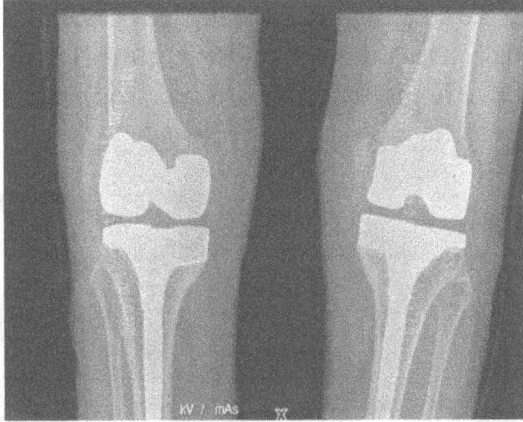

Figure 32: X-rays showing joint replacement components

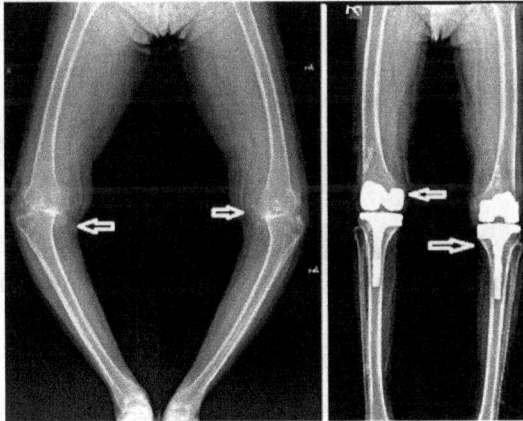

Figure 33: Radiograph showing a severe bow leg and straight legs after surgery

Case 11: 'Wheelchair to the Gym' - Hip Replacement for Rescue After Several Failed Fracture Surgeries

Forty-eight-year-old Kamala (name changed) met with a catastrophic road traffic accident three years ago and sustained double fractures in her right hip and thigh. This was initially treated with multiple surgeries in a nearby hospital where multiple screws and a rod were inserted in her hip and thigh bones, respectively.

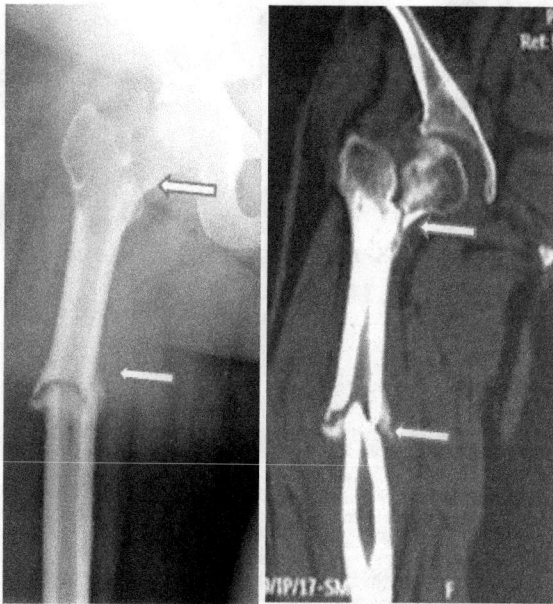

Figure 34: Double fractures and damaged hip joint

Unfortunately, within four weeks of this surgery, she developed an infection in her hip joint. Even after several antibiotics and surgical cleaning, the infection failed to settle. Eventually, her primary surgeon had to remove all the metal implants from her bone to control the infection spread even though the fractures weren't healed yet. She was left bed-bound for six months.

When I saw her, things did not look good. The fractures were not healed, the blood supply to the hip joint was impaired, the ball and socket joint was not functional, and she was bed-bound. We had to fix the fracture as well as deal with the damaged hip joint. A hip replacement with a long stem was performed.

Ceramic type hip implants were used as she was young; it was one lengthy surgery. Kamala had developed embolism [blood clot or air block] during surgery, which blocked the blood supply to her lungs. Still, the anaesthetists, cardiologists, and pulmonologists did an excellent job managing it.

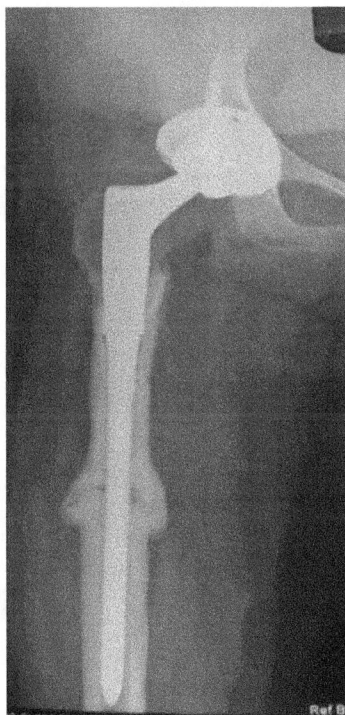

Figure 35: Long stem hip replacement to bridge the fracture

In about 12 weeks after surgery, the fracture was healed, and there was no pain seen in her hip. She resumed all her daily activities, and the last time I saw her, she was completely fine and had even started working out in a nearby fitness club.

7
ARTHRITIS IN
THE YOUNG

Summary:

Young patients can avoid joint replacement surgeries by adopting several alternative methods and surgeries other than joint replacements. If successful, these interventions can at least postpone the eventual total joint replacement surgery to an appropriate age.

Severe pain arises from the end-stage joint disease, usually in elderly patients. Having tried other alternatives, many settle for total joint replacement surgery. Although it may be successful, it is crucial to note that these procedures have a limited life span.

If performed at a younger age, the patients will require a more complicated revision of joint replacement during their lifetime.

Hence, total joint replacements are usually avoided in younger patients and are always seen as the last resort. However, sometimes, young patients will have no option but to undergo surgery as the pain limits their daily activities. Some of these procedures relieve pain and postpones the total joint replacements by a decade or more. Following are the commonly used options:

1. Arthroscopy
2. High tibial osteotomy
3. Partial or Unicondylar knee replacement

Arthroscopy

In athletes and young individuals, the use of surgical debridement as a treatment for osteoarthritis is controversial. Generally, arthroscopy is not recommended to patients with a primary diagnosis of symptomatic osteoarthritis. However, for those with meniscal tears, arthroscopic treatment may offer significant benefits.

One problem with this procedure is that it cannot address the real issue inside the knee — 'wear and tear.' As this procedure cannot restore the damaged cartilages, it will eventually fail. In recent times, this procedure is largely abandoned for primary arthritis of the knee.

High Tibial Osteotomy (HTO)

High Tibial Osteotomy is a commonly performed surgery in young patients suffering from knee pain. This surgery involves making a cut in the leg bone just below the knee joint and correcting the leg's alignment.

Correcting the knee's mechanical weight-bearing axis helps by relieving pressure from the arthritic portion of the joint and transferring it to an area of more normal cartilage. Restoration of the axis also prevents further deterioration of the affected part.

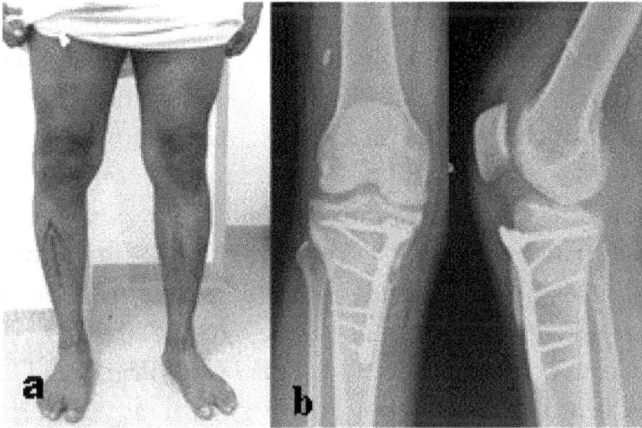

Figure 36: a) Mild bow leg deformity (Varus)of the right knee and b) Corrective high tibial osteotomy

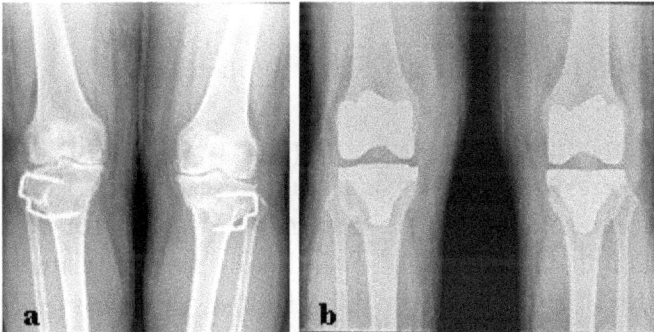

Figure 37: a) X-ray showing sever osteoarthritis of the knee, 15 years after the high tibial osteotomy and (b) eventual total knee replacement

This operation is for young patients if their knee involves some degree of deformity, such as a bowleg. Similar procedures can also be done if there is a knock-knee called valgus deformity [explored in chapter 3], but that is rare.

Lateral closing wedge osteotomy, medial open wedge osteotomy, and dome osteotomy are the common types of this procedure. HTO is contra-indicated if osteoarthritis has involved all the compartments of the knee, obese, severe deformities, and additional ligament injuries such as ACL tear. Statistics have shown that about 65% to 75% of patients were satisfied with the tibial osteotomy, even ten years after the operation. However, if the patient's weight is more than 1.32 times the ideal body weight, then survivorship decreases to 38% at five years and 19% at ten years.

Complications after High Tibial Osteotomy (HTO) are rare, but risks of infection, stiffness, and nerve injuries are possible. Results will deteriorate with time; it can be a decade or more. These patients may require a total knee replacement at that time, which will usually be an ideal age for a Total Knee Replacement.

Partial (Unicondylar) Knee Replacement

Unicondylar knee replacement also called unicompartmental or partial knee replacement (PKR), is a less invasive and more preservative option for younger patients with osteoarthritis. PKRs are associated with lesser surgical time, blood loss, transfusion, and rehabilitation period. Thus, the post-recovery rate is higher in PKR when compared to total knee replacements. Unicondylar knee replacement is suggested to those patients who suffer from significant pain in one compartment of the knee that does not respond to non-operative treatments.

However, this surgery is not advised for advanced knee disease, severe deformities such as inability to fold the knee beyond 90 degrees, bowing of more than 10 degrees, loose ligaments, and inability to straighten the knee entirely beyond 10 degrees.

If other compartments are involved, then partial knee replacement cannot be performed. It is also applicable for inflammatory arthritis like rheumatoid arthritis. Again, these results are poor in obese patients.

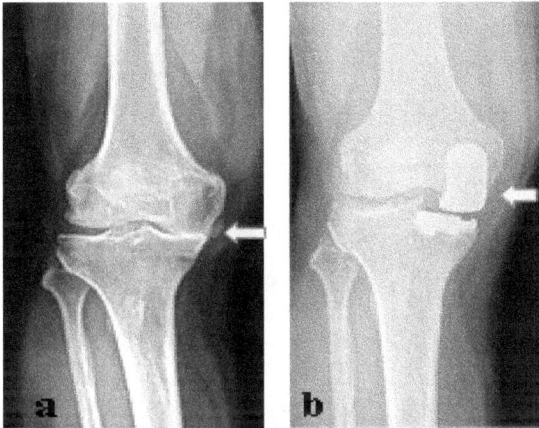

Figure 38: a) Narrowing of the gap on the inner compartment of the knee due to osteoarthritis b) Partial knee replacement

Partial knee replacements usually last for about 10 to 15 years. In a prospective follow-up study of 1,819 patients from the Finnish Arthroplasty Register, the overall 10-year Unicondylar knee replacement (UKR) survival was 73%. There was no difference in the patient-related outcomes compared to total knee replacements, but partial knee replacements last shorter.

Other than usual complications related to surgery, the most common mechanism of failure of partial knee replacements has been the loosening of the components with time (45%). They can also fail because of the progression of the osteoarthritis to the other compartments of the knee, polyethylene wear, technical and mechanical faults, osteoporosis, and some patients have unexplained pain.

Failed partial knee replacements usually require revision surgery, most likely a total knee replacement. Again, by then, most of the patients would have reached an appropriate age to undergo total knee replacement. Revision of a failed partial knee replacement to a primary total knee replacement is favorable compared to a revision knee replacement of a failed primary TKR.

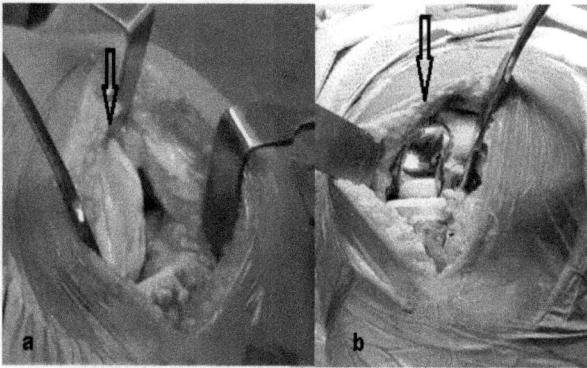

Figure 39: a) Partially worn-out cartilage of the knee b) Replaced with partial knee replacement

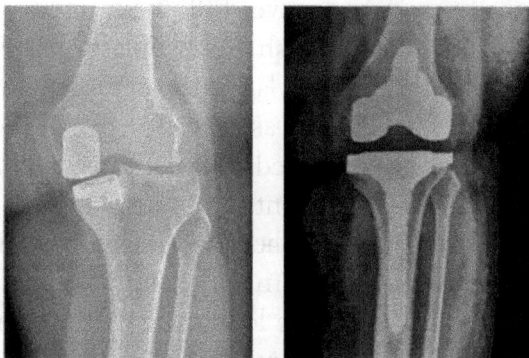

Figure 40: [Left] Failed partial knee replacement [Right] Revised total knee replacement

References:

1) Mohamad J. Halawi, Wael K. Barsoum: Unicondylar knee arthroplasty: Key concepts. J Clin Orthop Trauma. Jan-Mar 2017;8(1):11-13.

2) Amoako AO, Pujalte GG; Osteoarthritis in young, active, and athletic individuals. Clin Med Insights Arthritis Musculoskelet Disord. 2014 May 22;7:27-32.

3) Borus T, Thornhill T. Unicompartmental knee arthroplasty. J Am Acad Orthop Surg. 2008;16:9–18.

4) DeRogatis M, Anis HK, Sodhi N, Ehiorobo JO, Chughtai M, Bhave A, Mont MA. Non-operative treatment options for knee osteoarthritis. Ann Transl Med 2019;7(Suppl 7):S245.

5) Lucie Brosseau, Lucie Pelland, et al (2004) Efficacy of Aerobic Exercises For Osteoarthritis (part II): A Meta-analysis, Physical Therapy Reviews, 9:3, 125-145.

Case 12: Partial Knee Replacement to Rescue This Teacher

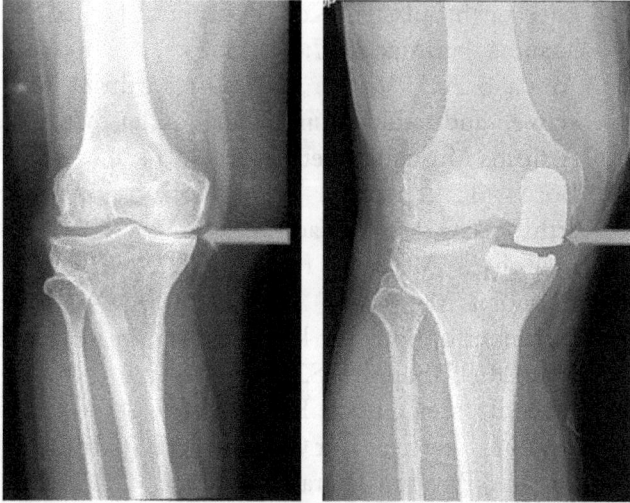

Figure 41: [Left]Narrowed joint space only half of the Joint
[Right] Partial knee replacement

Mrs Chethana (name changed), a 47-year-old teacher, had been suffering from severe pain in her right knee for more than four years. Her occupation demanded her to stand for hours together every day. After working the entire day, she used to find it extremely difficult to perform other activities back home. She underwent several treatments, including physiotherapy, administered three knee injections, and consumed all prescribed medications. However, none of them proved to be useful. The situation worsened over the days, and Chethana ended up dragging her legs while walking. Performing simple everyday activities became a task.

She had severe osteoarthritis on the inner part of her knee. Her knee was partially involved with the rest of the knee being still intact. Because her young age a partial knee replacement was considered appropriate as partial knee replacement replaces only the portion of the knee which is affected.

Unlike TKR, this operation does not involve many complications. A successful partial knee replacement will work for about 10 to 15 years. These patients will receive TKR, later when they are older.

Mrs Chethana finally underwent partial knee replacement. She recovered well and was discharged within three days. She was able to return to her work in six weeks. It is now about three years since her surgery, and she is full of energy and does all her activities without any pain.

Case 13: My Youngest Patient to Get a Total Knee Replacement (34-year-old)

Radha (name changed) is a young, brilliant software professional who, unfortunately, was a victim of juvenile rheumatoid arthritis. She started experiencing joint pain when she was just 19-years-old. She was being treated with rheumatoid medicines. Initially, the medications helped her to manage the pain but over the years, her state worsened, and she could hardly walk or sleep.

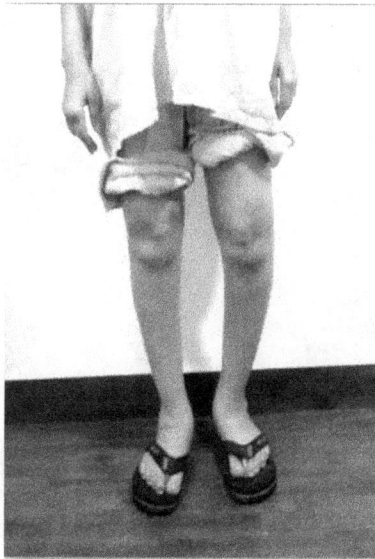

Figure 42: Bent knees because of juvenile rheumatoid arthritis

The doctors increased her dosage of rheumatoid medications, and she was given biologicals - a new class of strong rheumatoid medicines. Although this helped her for some time, the situation got bad overtime, and it also started interfering with her daily activities. It was at this moment that her rheumatologist suggested knee replacements.

When she was examined and considered for knee replacements, it was evident that she would need surgery and that it could greatly benefit her.

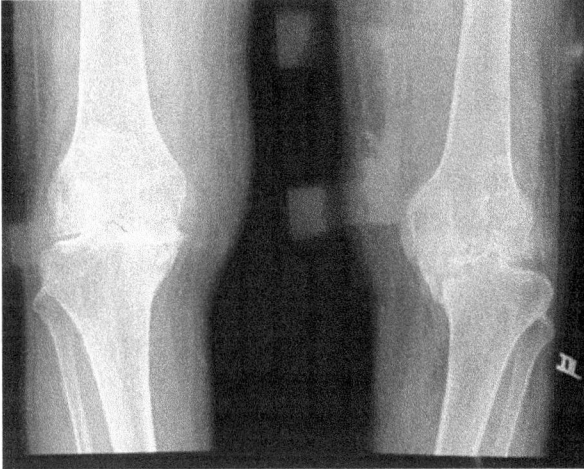

Figure 43: Both knee with severe arthritis showing complete obliteration of space

However, her age was not ideal for total joint replacement as it is sure to fail after a few years; most joint replacements last only for about 20 to 25 years at their best. As she is still in her 30s, she might be needing multiple revision surgeries going forward.

For context, revision surgeries are complicated, and the success rate is not that good. Avoiding joint replacement at a young age is one of the vital treatment goals for people of her age group. So, I sent her back to the rheumatologist and advised her to consult a physiotherapist and an orthotist.

We provided her with a weight relieving knee braces and several medications for a trial period of six months. However, the situation worsened as her pain and disability started affecting her, both physically and emotionally. She then got back to me and asked for a joint replacement surgery as she wanted to lead an active life.

Anyway, we operated on her, and she got both her knees replaced simultaneously. Because of her favourable young age, she recovered very quickly.

Within about six weeks, she was back at all her activities. Patients who have juvenile rheumatoid arthritis may need total knee replacements at an early age compared to osteoarthritis. In general, joint replacements last longer in rheumatoid arthritis patients because of the lesser physical activity these patients can perform.

Radha says she has got a new lease of life. All we can do is hope that her joints last much longer than 20 years.

Case 14: This Young Actor Who Underwent Both Hip Replacements

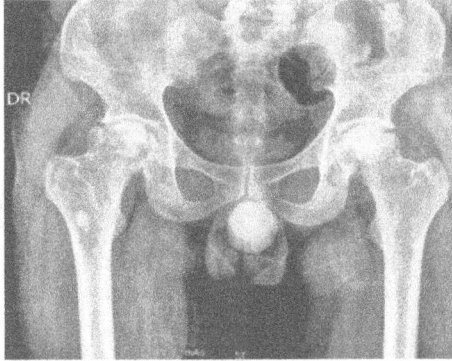

**Figure 44: X -ray prior to the surgery
showing damaged, uneven
ball and socket joint**

Mr. Vinod (name changed), a young budding actor visited my clinic back in May 2012, complaining of severe pain in his right hip. He had been experiencing severe pain in that hip for more than three years. Besides affecting his career, the pain also restricted him from performing basic daily activities.

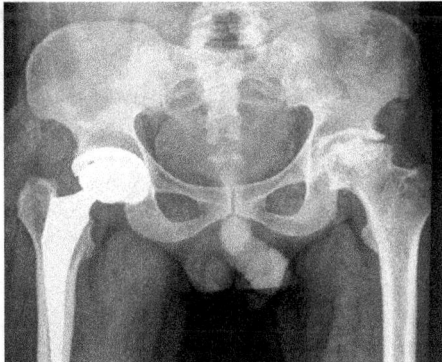

**Figure 45: After one (right) hip
replacement**

Called 'avascular necrosis' of the hip, the blood supply to the hip is blocked due to a variety of reasons in this condition. The exact cause of this problem may remain unknown in many of these patients.

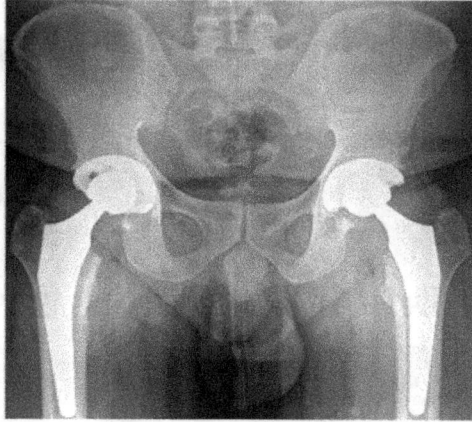

Figure 46: After both total hip replacements

Vinod underwent total hip replacement surgery on his right hip and recovered surprisingly well. However, he had to return to the hospital after three years after experiencing severe pain in his other hip. The X-ray report showed severe arthritis in the left hip, and he had to undergo another hip replacement. He is currently back in all his activities and is going about his career without any pain. The acquaintances he made post his hip surgery cannot even make out that he has had hip surgery.

Case 15: She Needed a Hip Replacement Before She Could Deliver Her Baby

Mrs. Swathi (name changed), a young lady in her early 30s had consulted me along with her husband regarding her hip dysplasia condition. For context, in this condition, the hip joints are not well developed since childhood, and the person is seen limping all the time. Swathi had been suffering from the same condition, and her pain had worsened with age.

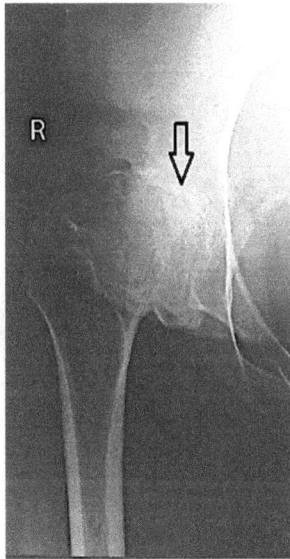

Figure 47: Hip not developed properly by birth and now lost its shape

The young couple was planning for a baby, and as per their previous consultation with a gynecologist, given Swathi's condition, she wouldn't be able to widen her legs during the time of the delivery; this could end up being a major complication in her pregnancy. It was a difficult decision to make. I could not easily advise her to undergo a total hip replacement because of her young age. But she was suffering from severe pain and also this issue was hindering her social life and their family planning.

After a lengthy discussion and counselling, she decided to go for hip replacement. We had to consider several factors related to a replacement including a suitable material. Metal on metal type resurfacing was not an option as the metal ions could end up having adverse effects on the baby. We decided to go for a ceramic hip replacement because this is the most inert material for a replacement. The surgery was a success, and she recovered quite well.

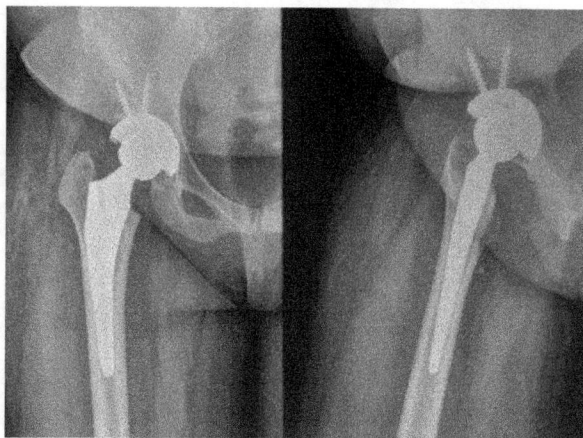

Figure 48: Pictures of the hip radiographs showing total hip replacement

Within three weeks of her surgery, she travelled abroad and joined her husband. To her and her husband's delight she recovered very quickly. She started going to the gym and even started playing tennis in just about six months, post-surgery. She conceived the very next year, and they were blessed with a healthy baby girl. Yes, it was a normal delivery.

8
TOTAL KNEE REPLACEMENT

Summary:

Knee replacement is performed during these three conditions –

- **The pain is severe**
- **Daily activities are being affected**
- **All the other options are exhausted.**

In these cases, an artificial implant is fixed inside the knee joint to relieve pain and restore mobility.

Total Knee Replacement, also known as Total Knee Arthroplasty, is one of the most successful and cost-effective interventions in modern medicine. The number of procedures performed each year has increased tremendously in the last decade, and it has been projected to increase further in the coming years.

Many studies have documented survival rates over 95% after 15 years of follow-up. The goals of knee replacement surgery are relieving pain, restoring mobility, enabling activities of daily living, correcting the alignment and deformities.

When Do You Need a Knee Replacement?

Knee replacement is commonly performed in the elderly population to relieve severe pain. The primary indication is osteoarthritis, which accounts for over 90% of total knee replacements, followed by rheumatoid arthritis. All forms of arthritis and other joint diseases can lead to severe damage to the joints, making replacement surgery a need — here, the cartilage is severely damaged, resulting in severe pain and affecting all daily activities. This stage is called end-stage joint disease.

Remember, not all patients with arthritis need surgery. The majority of them can be managed without surgery, even though they are not entirely curable. You should consider a knee replacement only if you are one or more things mentioned below.

- Aged above 60 years
- Severe pain
- Daily activities are impaired
- Taking too many painkillers
- Experiencing severe pain in the night
- Other forms of treatment have been tried and failed.

Not all the patients who undergo surgery fulfil all the above criteria. For example, someone much younger than 60 years, but severely affected by knee pain, may also be considered for surgery.

In rheumatoid arthritis, patients usually suffer from the involvement of multiple joints at a younger age. Due to the crippling nature of this disease, surgery is performed even in younger patients. However, there should be evidence of severe damage in a standing radiograph(X-rays) of the knee, in case of younger patients. The doctor will rule out other sources of leg pain, such as pain radiating from the spine or hip.

Other factors like body weight and medical fitness to surgery are also important. Generally, patients who are young and obese have less favourable long-term results.

When Can't You Have a Knee Replacement?

These situations are called medical contraindications. In these conditions, you are not a candidate for joint replacement surgery despite suffering from severe pain.

• You should not undergo surgery if you are suffering from an infection of a joint. If an artificial joint is placed in the presence of an infection, the operation will fail catastrophically within a matter of a few days to weeks.

• Avoid a joint replacement surgery if you are currently suffering from an infection anywhere else in the body because this can spread to your artificial knees.

• Total knee replacement won't function properly and will fail rapidly if the muscles of that joint are weak. Poliomyelitis or other paralytic conditions, for example.

• If you are suffering from decreased blood supply to the affected joint, healing of the surgical wound may be impaired.

• You should not have an operation if you are suffering from a severe illness, which may prevent you from having safe anaesthesia.

Preparations for Surgery (24 hours before surgery)

Usually, you are admitted a day before the surgery for general evaluation. In some cases, this can also be done a week before, in a specially designed preoperative assessment clinic. If you are fit and all the evaluations are completed, you can get admitted on the same day of your surgery.

Here, you will need assessment by an anaesthetist, general physician, or an internist. You may also require a cardiologist to see you. You will then receive a batch of blood tests, an ECG, an Echocardiogram, and a chest X-ray.

How is a Knee Replacement Done?

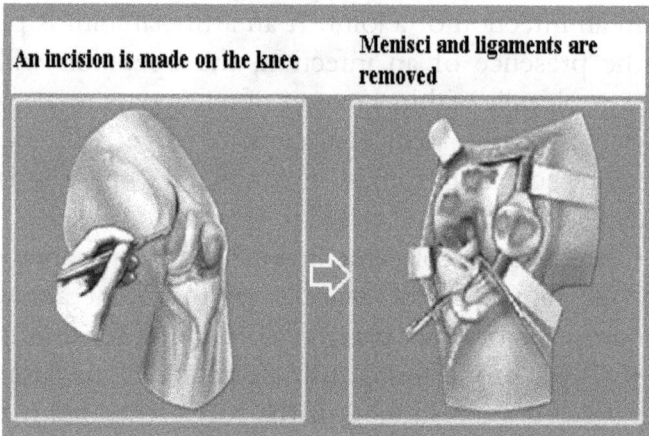

| An incision is made on the knee | Menisci and ligaments are removed |

Figure 49: Surgical steps of the knee replacement

Knee replacement is performed under the influence of anaesthesia. Depending on your general health, the anaesthetist will decide whether to administer general or spinal anaesthesia. The procedure is not done under local anaesthesia as it covers very little area; it is insufficient for this surgery.

You may also be administered epidural anaesthesia, femoral block, or adductor block, which will help you to control the pain for the following two days after surgery. A variety of preparations take place prior to the surgery. The cleaning, sterilizing, and covering you with sterile drapes - all this takes about 20 minutes. Then the surgeon, along with his team, also gets into complete sterile drapes.

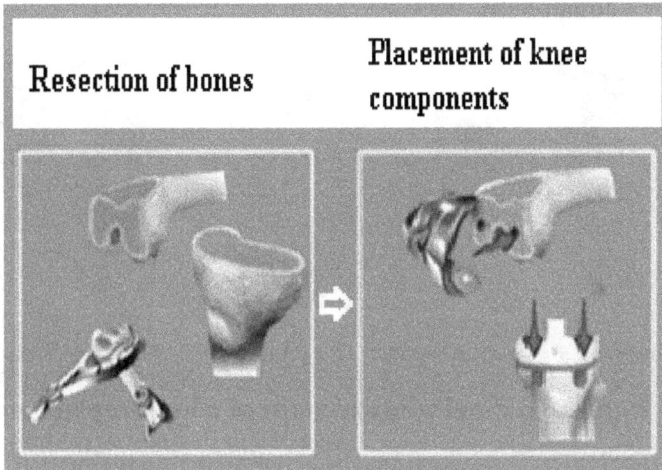

Figure 50: Surgical steps of the knee replacement

Surgery is performed with a midline longitudinal cut of about 8cm to 10cm on your knee. The surgeon will expose the bones of your knee, following which the thigh bone called 'femur', leg bone called 'tibia', and the kneecap called 'patella' are visualized. The sizes of your bones are also measured. Mechanical instruments and jigs are used to make precise cuts on these bones to remove the bone's worn-out parts.

Bones are cut in such a way that components are correctly fixed. Components of all sizes will be available every time a knee replacement is done. The surgeon will now make sure that your leg's alignment is straight, and the ligaments on both sides of the knee are balanced.

A trial of your knee movements and other parameters are checked with a trial prosthesis. If everything is satisfactory, then the final components are fixed on your bone using bone cement.

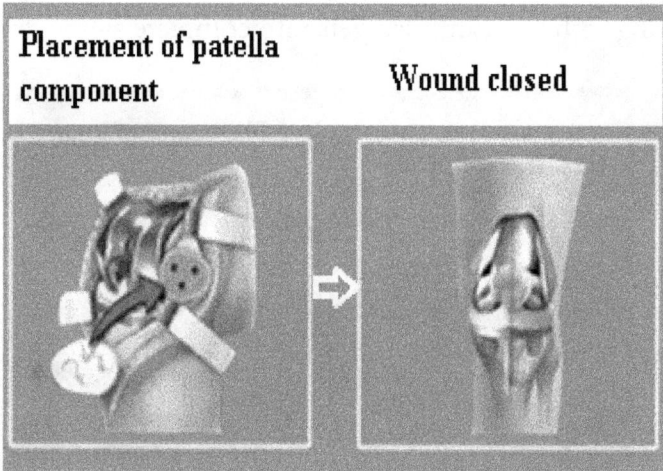

Figure 51: Final surgical steps of a knee replacements

Cement usually hardens in about 15 minutes, after which the wound is stitched layer by layer. The wound's dressing is not disturbed for at least two days.

After the surgery, patients will be shifted to a recovery area for a couple of hours for observation and then moved to the ward. While most patients do not require intensive care, those who undergo both knee replacements and those who suffer from other severe medical conditions might be shifted to an intensive care unit for monitoring. These patients will be allowed to drink and eat once they recover from general anaesthesia. They are also taught simple bedside exercises once they can sit up.

Point to note here is that patients recover at their own

pace and should not push themselves beyond their limits. For instance, while some patients may be able to walk on the same day, the majority will start walking only the next day.

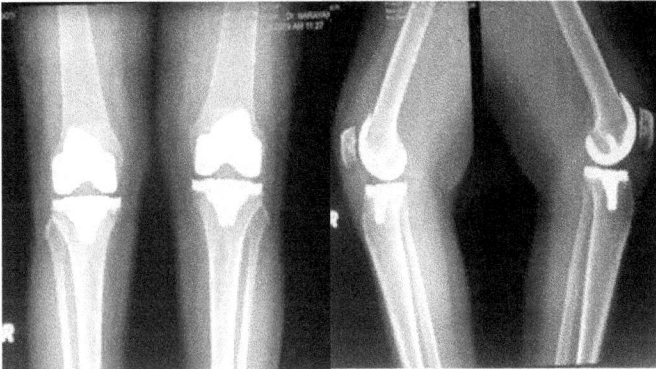

Figure 52: X rays from the front and sides after simultaneous total knee replacement

References:

1. Narayan Hulse: Total knee replacement in arthritis - Current Concepts. Chapter 9. Frontiers in Arthritis, Ashish Anand (ed). 2017, Vol 1, 105-127.

2. Liu HW, Gu WD, Xu NW, Sun JY: Surgical approaches in total knee arthroplasty: a meta-analysis comparing the midvastus and subvastus to the medial peripatellar approach. J Arthroplasty. 2014 Dec;29(12):2298-304.

3. Keblish PA: The lateral approach to the valgus knee. Surgical technique and analysis of 53 cases with over two-year follow-up evaluation. Clin Orthop Relat Res. 1991 Oct;(271):52-62.

4. Scuderi GR, Tenholder M, Capeci C: Surgical approaches in mini-incision total knee arthroplasty. Clin Orthop Relat Res. 2004 Nov;(428):61-7.

Case 16: Severe Bow-Legs: Can It Be Corrected?

'Will my bowlegs be corrected post-surgery?', 'Will it be partially corrected or fully corrected?' — These are the questions that are generally asked by patients who are considering a knee replacement. Although bowlegs are common with osteoarthritis, many develop only a mild deformity.

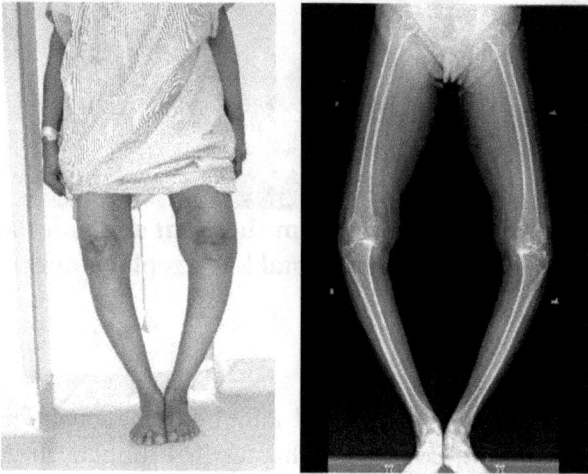

Figure 53: Bow-legs before knee replacements

Mrs. Savitri (name changed), a 65-year-old housewife, had been suffering from knee pain and bowlegs for more than ten years. She was quite sceptical about getting a knee replacement until she visited her son in the USA and got acquainted with a family doctor and another patient who had undergone the same surgery.

Convinced by the benefits of knee replacements, Savitri came back to India and underwent a knee replacement. It was performed using computer navigation. Preoperatively, the bowing in each leg was about 40 degrees and post-surgery, they were completely straightened. A stemmed knee replacement was used because of soft bones and the large correction.

Mrs. Savitri was pleased about her surgery and is now able to perform all activities on her own while staying pain- free.

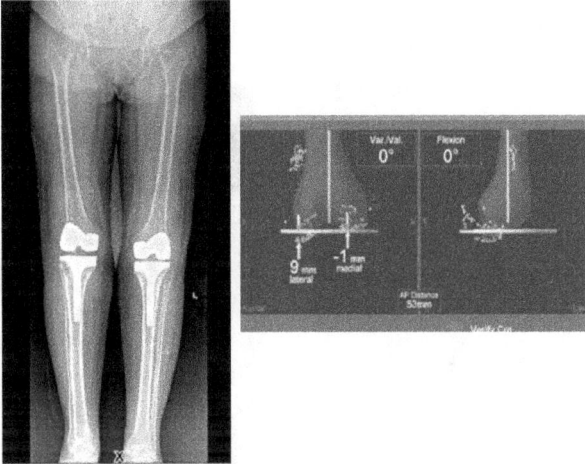

Figure 54: Radiograph after surgery and records of the computer navigation

Case 17: 'Wind-Swept Knee'- Even Though She Couldn't Stand, Her Ayurvedic Doctor Dissuaded Her TKR for Six Years.

'Windswept deformity' is a rare condition of the knee where both the knees are bent to the same side — Bowleg on one side and a knock-knee on the other (figure 55).

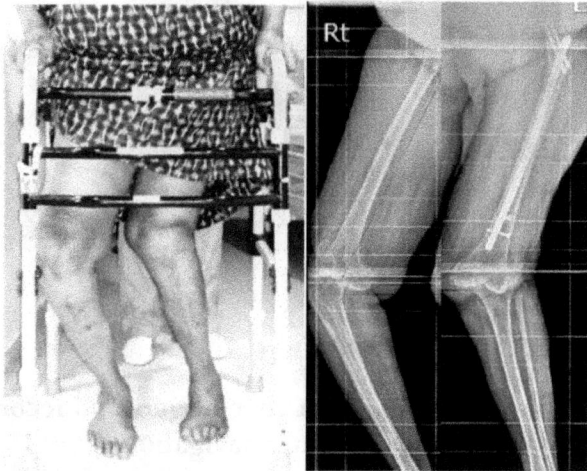

Figure 55: Walking with a frame and bent knees

Mrs. Shah (name changed), a 55-year-old lady, had rheumatoid arthritis for over ten years. Pain and immobility had affected her immensely, and she could barely walk even with the help of a walker.

One day, she suffered a fall in the washroom and sustained a fracture in her right hip. This incident complicated the treatment of the already existing severe arthritis in her knees.

We treated her left hip fracture by surgically inserting a rod. Although she recovered from the hip fracture within six months, her bad knees gave her a tough time while walking around. In my opinion, she should have undergone both knee replacements much earlier; this could have actually prevented her fall.

Mrs. Shah was not very keen on undergoing a knee replacement even at this point. All thanks to the traditional medical practitioner that she had trusted for many years; he had continuously discouraged her from undergoing a knee replacement.

Finally, as she could not bear the pain anymore, she underwent both knee replacements. She was extremely satisfied with the surgery and enjoyed her new-found mobility. Within a month, she sent me a video of her walking independently at home. Following this, eight of her friends and relatives also underwent knee replacements.

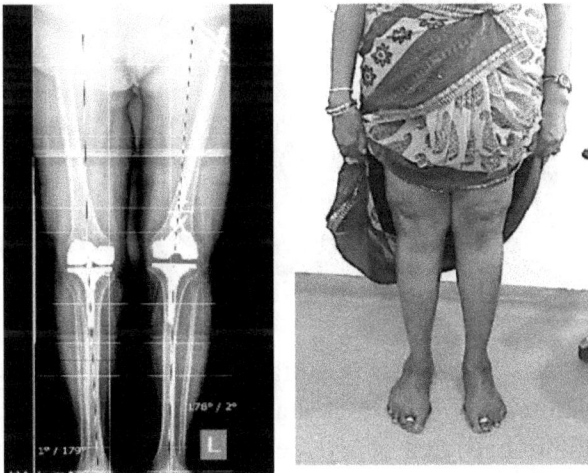

Figure 56: Straightened knees after surgery

Mrs. Shah has always been a happy lady. She used to cook for the entire family while sitting on a chair next to the kitchen stand, before the operation! Her joyful nature helped her get through her sufferings.

Case 18: He Grew 8 cm Taller After the Knee Replacements!

Mr. Ravi (name changed) is a 49-year-old pharmacist working in a government dispensary. He was born with a medical condition that stunted his growth and resulted in severe bowing of his knees (figure 57). Although he underwent multiple surgeries to correct the deformities in his childhood, nothing really worked.

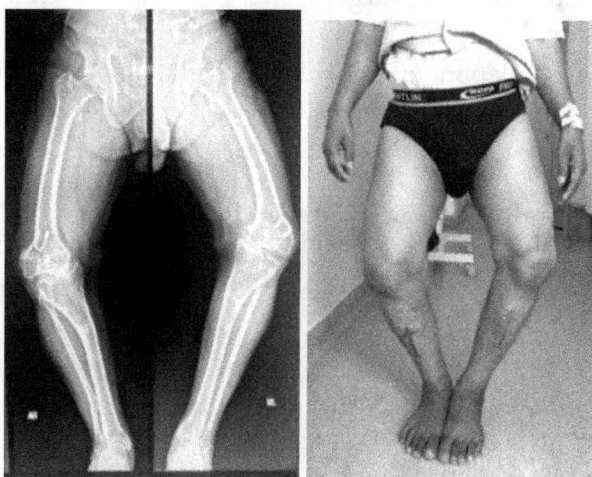

Figure 57: Bow-legs before surgery

He was about 4.9 feet tall; bowing of his legs also contributed to his short stature. In the preceding two years, he had developed severe pain and difficulty in walking. Although he underwent multiple physiotherapy sessions and took loads of medications, his quality of life deteriorated significantly, and he finally considered a knee replacement.

Since this is a medically complicated case, normal techniques of a knee replacement were difficult to employ. In his case, routine straight instruments could not be passed inside the bones because of the multiple bents in the leg bones.

It was also difficult to calculate the angles manually at various points on the leg. Hence a computer navigated knee replacement was necessary.

Surgery was done in two stages at a five-day interval. His leg alignment was corrected using complex calculations with the help of the computer navigation system (figure 58).

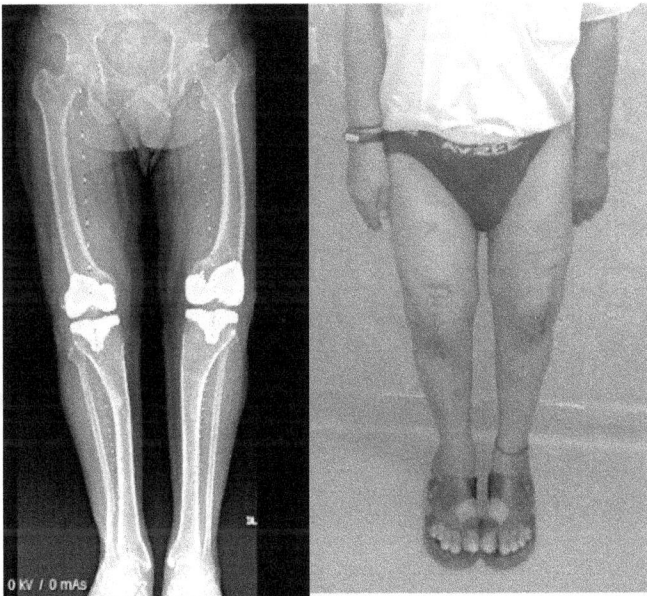

Figure 58: After surgery

As he was very enthusiastic and cheerful during the entire process, he took the rehabilitation phase very positively and started showing signs of recovery within four to six weeks. He even returned to work after six weeks. To everybody's pleasant surprise, he had grown taller by about 8 cm and was walking straight!

9
TOTAL HIP REPLACEMENT

Summary:
Total hip replacement is the second commonly performed joint replacement surgery, after total knee replacement. This is usually indicated for those with severe pain in their hip joints and a variety of arthritic and related conditions.

Hip replacement is one of the most successful orthopaedic interventions, and hence, it is described as 'The operation of the 20th century'.

Following all the developments in the modern total hip replacement techniques, especially the one by Sir John Charnley in the 1960s, millions of people have undergone hip surgeries all over the globe.

This operation is thus regarded as the most exceptional medical intervention of the 20th century, taking into account the fact that these developments have improved the quality of life in millions of patients.

Who Needs Hip Replacements?

Most of the diseases affecting the hip joint can damage the hip cartilage progressively. If the cartilage damage is causing severe pain, affecting the daily activities and is not relieved by non-operative treatment, then the person has to undergo a hip replacement surgery.

The general perspective is that replaced hips can be in good condition for about 20 years, and hence it is also preferred that total hip arthroplasty be done only in patients older than 60 years. At this age, the physical demands on the prosthesis tend to be fewer, and the longevity of the replaced hip approaches the life expectancy of the patient.

The most common medical conditions requiring hip replacement are:

1. Osteoarthritis
2. Rheumatoid arthritis
3. Secondary osteoarthritis due to congenital dysplasia hip
4. Trauma
5. Paget's disease
6. Avascular necrosis of the hip
7. Ankylosing spondylitis, and many more

When Can't You Have a Hip Replacement?

These situations are called medical contraindications. You are not a candidate for joint replacement surgery despite having severe pain if you are currently suffering from an infection in the hip or anywhere else in the body.

If you still go ahead with the surgery, the infection might spread to your artificial hips, and the operation might catastrophically fail within a few days to weeks.

Total hip replacement might also fail if the muscles of that particular joint are fragile (poliomyelitis or other paralytic conditions, for instance).

Secondly, you should not have an operation if you are suffering from a severe illness which may prevent you from having safe anaesthesia.

Preparations for Surgery (24 Hours Before Surgery)

The preparations remain similar to the procedure that was discussed in the knee replacement surgery in chapter 8.

Technique of Hip Replacement

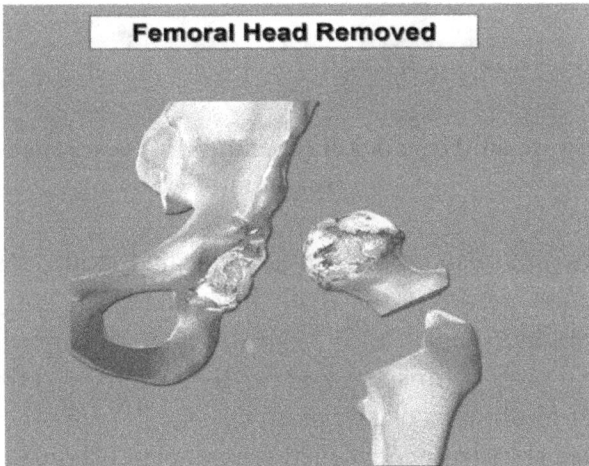

Figure 59: Femoral head (ball of the hip joints) removed

Regional or general anaesthesia – Both are reliable options for hip replacement. For this surgery, a cut of about 10cm- 12cm long is made on the side of the hip joint. The size and the site of the cut are solely dependent on the type of surgical approach, body weight, and also the complexity of the case—doctors visualize the hip joint using this incision.

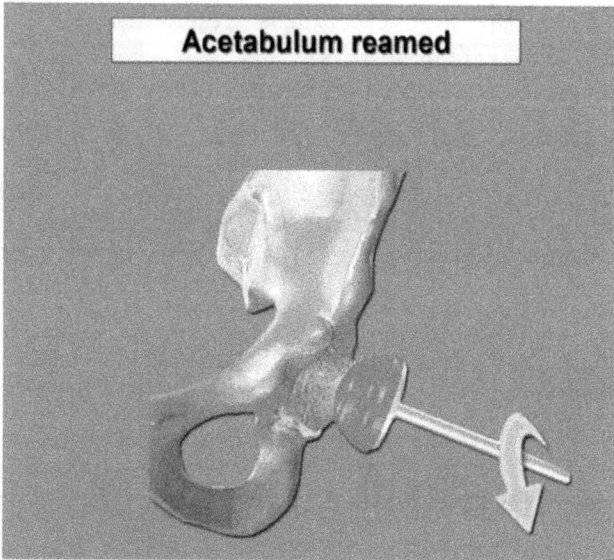

Figure 60: Hip socket (acetabulum) is scraped using reamers

Then the ball of the hip is dislocated from its socket. Surgeons remove the ball by making a cut at an appropriate angle and length using a surgical saw. Unnecessary soft tissues and debris are removed from the socket to obtain a clear vision.

Special instruments called reamers are used to prepare this new socket following which a trial is done using an appropriately same sized test–prosthesis. If satisfactory, a socket is fixed in the hip using bone cement or screws or simply a press-fit depending on the technique employed.

The upper end of the thigh bone is then prepared using other specific instruments. During this procedure, the hollow bone is scrapped to shape the center of the thigh bone to accommodate the femoral stem.

A trial stem with a ball on its top end is placed in the thigh bone, and surgeons manoeuvre it into the socket. He confirms the length of the leg, stability, and movement of the hip joint. At this stage, further refinement can be made by changing the size of the components. Once satisfactory, all the parts are placed back. Like the socket, stem can also be placed in the thigh bone with or without cement.

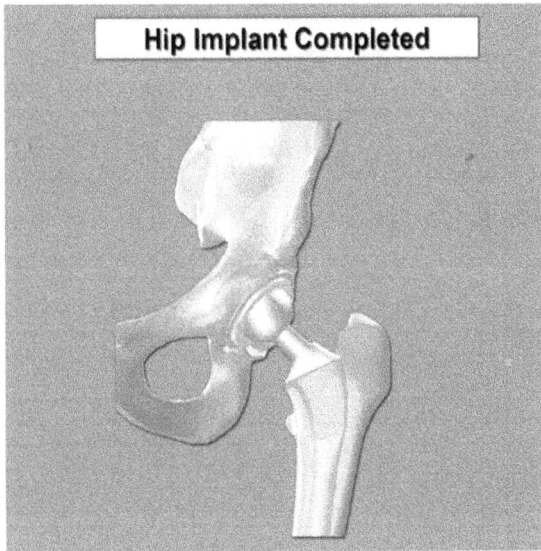

Figure 61: Hip prosthesis implanted

The surgical wounds are stitched layer by layer, and the dressing stays untouched for a couple of days. After the surgery, the patient is shifted to a recovery area for a couple of observational hours and then moved to the ward.

Like knee replacement surgery, most patients will not require intensive care post the hip replacement surgery. However, patients suffering from other medical conditions may be shifted to an intensive care unit for monitoring.

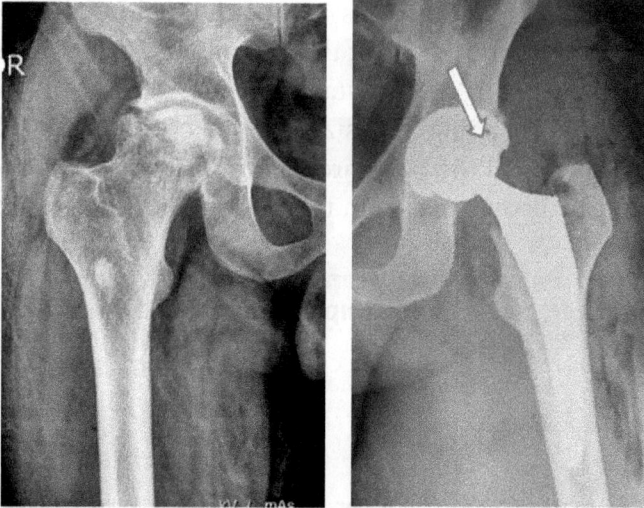

Figure 62: X-ray of the hip before and after surgery

References:

1) Learmonth ID, Young C, Rorabeck C: The operation of the century: total hip replacement. Lancet. 2007 Oct 27;370(9597):1508-19.

2) Hilal Maradit Kremers, Dirk R Larson, Cynthia S Crowson: Prevalence of Total Hip and Knee Replacement in the United States. J Bone Joint Surg Am. 2015.

3) Petis S, Howard JL, Lanting BL, Vasarhelyi EM: Surgical approach in primary total hip arthroplasty: anatomy, technique, and clinical outcomes. Can J Surg. 2015 Apr;58(2):128-39.

Case 19: The Scientist Needed a New Hip to Continue His Research

This scientist, who currently in his 50s, had met with a major accident when he was 42-year-old and since then, he had been experiencing some pain and difficulty in his left hip. Initially, he was able to manage the pain by reducing his physical activities and consuming painkillers occasionally. However, his pain only got worse over time. Instead of consulting a doctor right away, he increased his painkiller consumption.

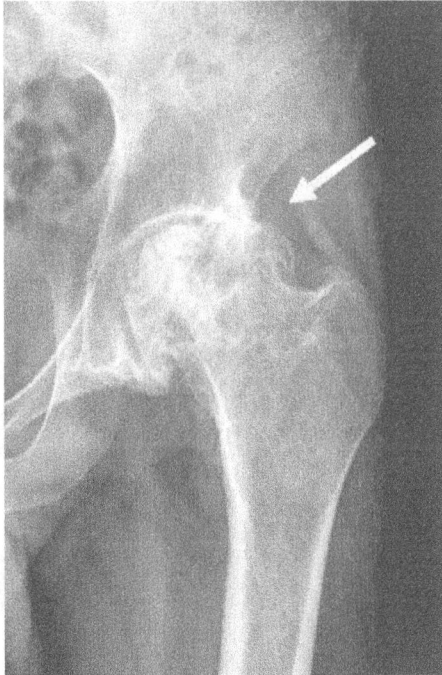

Figure 63: Damaged hip joint

By the time he approached me, he was in a lot of pain and was using a crutch to walk. He was completely unable to use his left leg. The X-rays revealed a damaged hip joint (figure 63).

He underwent a routine Total Hip Replacement surgery [the uncemented type (figure 64)]. The scientist was able to recover quickly because of his good health and general understanding. He was discharged within three days and was dependent on the stick during the initial days of surgery. On day 14, when he visited the hospital to get his stitches removed, he was walking independently. Following that, in less than four weeks, he was back at work continuing his research.

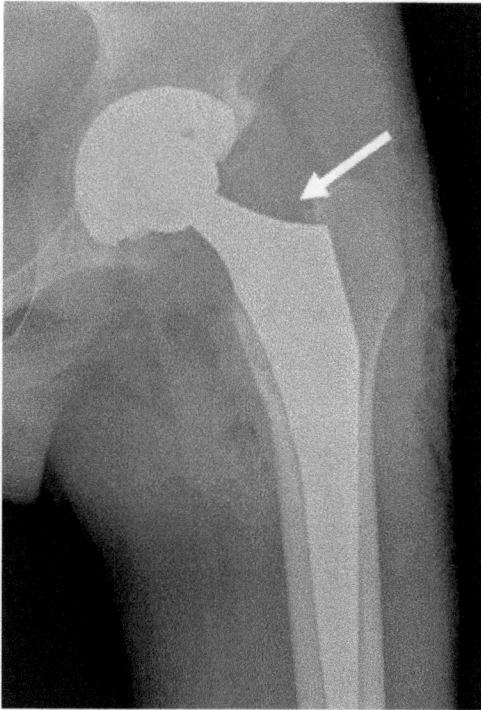

Figure 64: Radiograph after total hip replacement

Case 20: He Could Not Even Sit for Ten Years as His Hips Were Immovable

Thirty-year-old Raman (name changed) was suffering from an arthritic condition called 'ankylosing spondylitis'; this condition usually runs in families. Hips and spine are the main targets, and there is no proven cure to this condition, yet. Raman had been suffering from severe pain in his hips and spine for almost ten years.

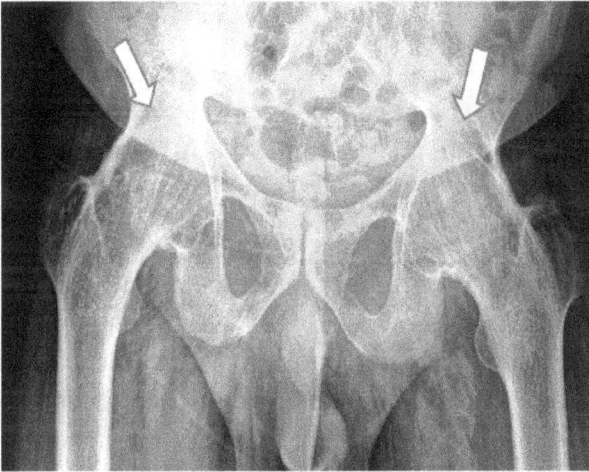

Figure 65: Arrows showing the fused hip joints showing no demarcation between the ball and socket

Due to this condition, his hip bones were fused together, rendering the entire joint immobile. For context, the hip joint is necessary to bend down the torso, and without this, it is not only impossible to sit on the floor but also on the chair.

This young man could never sit on a chair, commode, or even travel by car. Even during his visits to the hospital, he had to sit upright for the entire journey of 800 km.

Imagine how difficult this could have been! He could only stand or lie down; he managed to walk slowly. To add on, he always had to stand while eating and even while using the washroom.

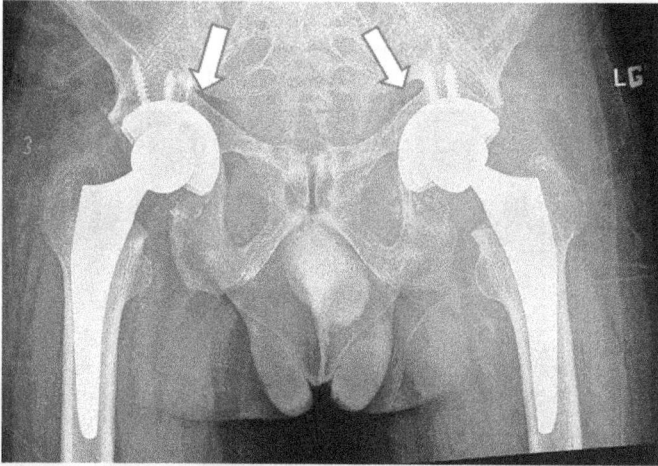

Figure 66: Both hip replacements in good position

Surgically, the correction was extremely challenging and also technically demanding. As there was no demarcation between the ball and socket, it wasn't easy to place the components in the correct position. However, the surgery was completed successfully. He underwent his left hip replacement first.

During the first week post-surgery, he faced several problems. One of them was the inability to eat or drink — he could neither sit (because of the immobility of the unoperated hip) nor stand (because of the surgical pain in the other operated hip.)

Hence the second hip was also operated after five days. The following day after the second surgery, everyone around him was literally in tears to see him sitting on the edge of the bed for the first time in ten years. He also walked a few steps with the help of a physiotherapist. To everybody's surprise, he recovered quickly and was comfortable doing all activities on his own.

For a surgeon, although such cases are incredibly challenging, it is satisfying to the core.

10
OTHER JOINT REPLACEMENTS

Summary:
  For those suffering from severe pain in other joints such as shoulder, elbow or ankle, surgical replacements are available. These procedures have been performed for many years now, however, they are not as popular as the knee and hip replacements. Partial joint replacements are also available for younger patients.

Total Shoulder Replacement

Our shoulders can be a victim of several disorders. It is a very complex joint and is involved in a wide range of movements associated with our hands. However, when it comes to joint replacement surgeries, total shoulder replacement isn't as popular as knee and hip replacements.

Shoulder is a non-weight bearing joint and when it comes to the disorders associated with it, many patients usually manage their pain without having to undergo a surgery.

That said, over the last three decades, total shoulder replacement has evolved as a fine operation and it has been a boon to those suffering from severe shoulder pain. Total shoulder replacement is often suggested to patients with osteoarthritis and inflammatory arthropathies such as rheumatoid arthritis.

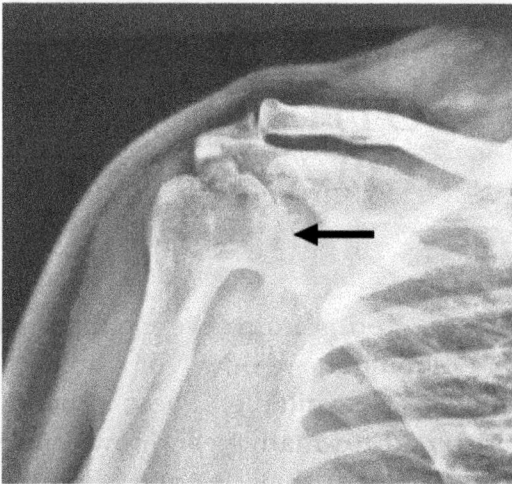

Figure 67: Shoulder arthritis with decreased joint space

Although total shoulder replacement is good for pain relief, it doesn't make way for full range of movements; many patients will not be able to achieve over the head movement of the arm.

Additionally, total shoulder replacements fail early if the muscles in the shoulder, the 'rotator cuff', is weak or ruptured. The results of shoulder arthroplasty also vary depending on the underlying diagnosis, the joint's condition, the soft tissues at the time of surgery, and the type of reconstruction performed.

However, the results of shoulder arthroplasty in primary osteoarthritis are satisfactory in majority of the patients. 90% of the individuals report an improvement in the pain; the average elevation among these patients is usually over 135 degrees.

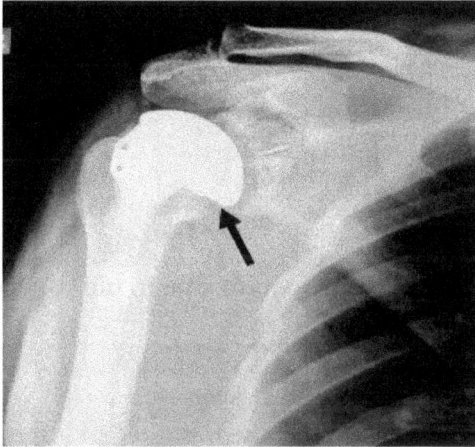

Figure 68: Total shoulder replacement

Reverse Shoulder Arthroplasty

When the shoulder joint develops painful wear and tear due to the torn rotator cuff muscles, reverse shoulder replacement is a reasonable option. This condition is referred to as 'cuff tear arthropathy'.

In this technique, the direction of the ball and socket are reversed. Meaning, the original concave-shaped socket is replaced by a metal ball and the original ball is replaced by a metal/polythene socket. This new direction enables the nearby muscle 'deltoid' to take over the function of the torn rotator cuff muscle.

Patients gain good control over the shoulder movements due to the semi constrained nature of the implant and an improved deltoid lever arm. Unlike, traditional total shoulder arthroplasty, reverse shoulder arthroplasty is less likely to have early failures.

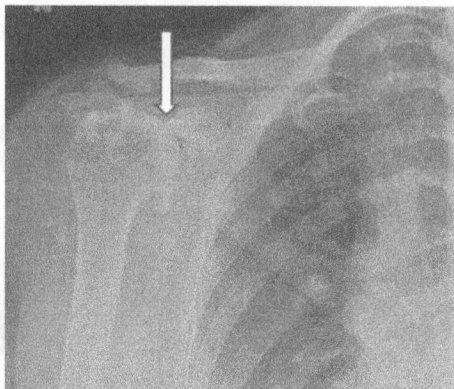

Figure 69: Arthritic joint due to old rotator cuff tear

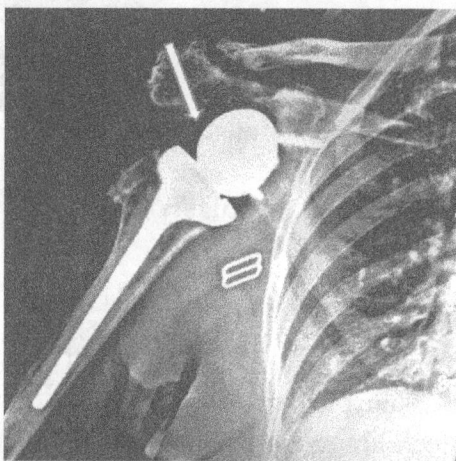

Figure 70: Picture after reverse shoulder replacement

The main indication for reverse shoulder arthroplasty is cuff-tear arthropathy. Reverse shoulder arthroplasty is also occasionally performed in cases of some types of fractures, revision surgeries, after resection of tumors, and massive shoulder muscles (cuff) tears even without arthritis.

Total Elbow Replacement

Compared to the hip and knee joints, the elbow joint is relatively small and is rarely affected by osteoarthritis and other arthritic diseases. The elbow's stability depends greatly on ligamentous integrity.

As I mentioned earlier, the elbow replacements are performed in fewer numbers when compared to the hip and knees.

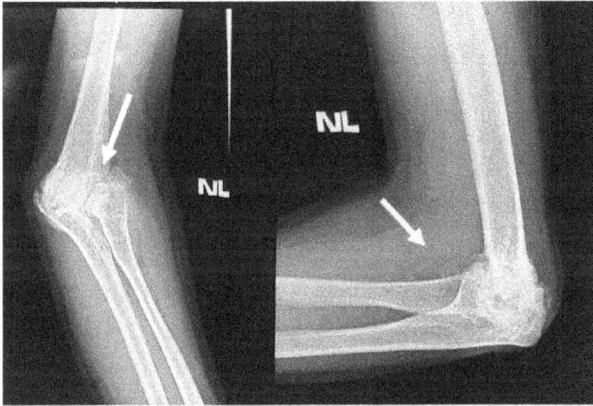

Figure 71: Arthritic elbow

Interestingly, the overall success rate of total elbow replacement is best in patients with inflammatory arthritis and also the elderly patients with acute distal humerus fractures. The results are not so good for patients with posttraumatic osteoarthritis.

The common complications associated with elbow arthroplasty include infection, loosening, wear, triceps weakness, and ulnar neuropathy. Once there is a requirement for revision surgery, the bone augmentation techniques provide a reasonable outcome.

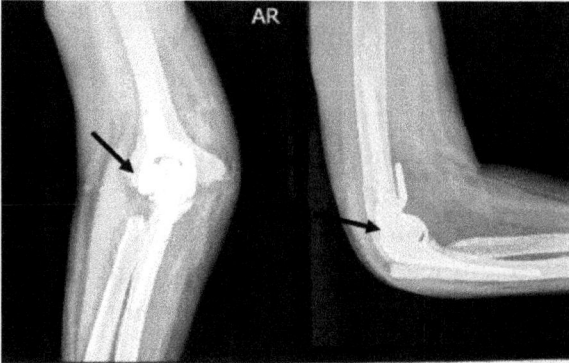

Figure 72: X-ray after elbow replacement

Total Ankle Replacement

This is one of the rarely performed joint replacement surgeries. Total ankle replacement was earlier considered inferior to ankle fusion due to its poor results. However, newer designs have shown improved clinical outcomes. Even though the controversy still exists, this procedure is performed commonly in elderly patients with inflammatory and other arthritic conditions.

Ankle replacement will function best in patients who are less active and not obese. But the prosthesis may get loose with time and may require complex revision or fusion of the ankle joint.

For instance, recent studies have shown as high as 90% of total ankle replacements to be still intact, even five years after surgery. However, it is also shown that this number drops to about 80% at around eight years after surgery.

Furthermore, complications after an ankle replacement are high if the patient has diabetes, poor blood circulation, or if there is a misalignment of the ankle due to previous fractures.

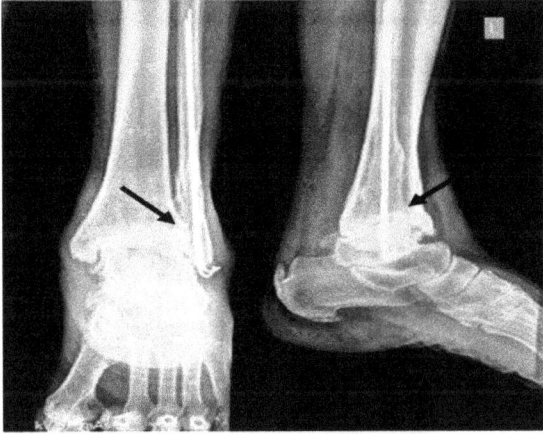

**Figure 73: Damaged ankle
due to an old fracture**

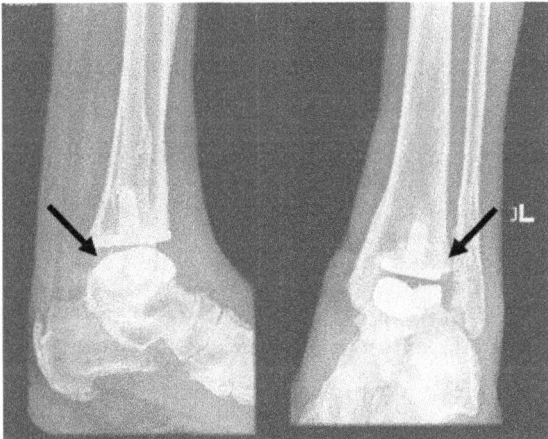

Figure 74: After total ankle replacement

Partial Knee Replacements (PKR)

This is described in the chapter 'Arthritis in The Young'.

Hip Resurfacing

Hip resurfacing in its current form is largely abandoned all over the world. This option is less favored because of the high risk of complications and early failure. This procedure has also fallen into disrepute over the years because of metal debris causing metal ions in the body, resulting in painful tumor-like swellings around the hip, fracture neck femur, and other complications.

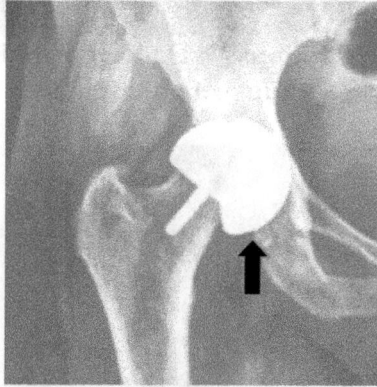

Figure 75: Failed hip resurfacing with the socket dislodged from its place

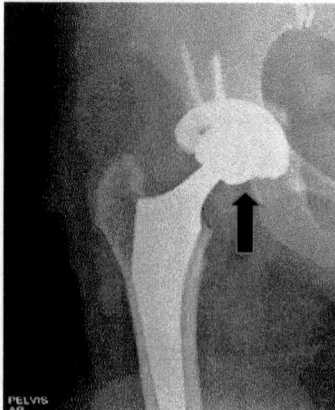

Figure 76: Revised to a total hip replacement

If that's on the negative end, hip resurfacing does have the advantage of bone preservation on the femur (thigh bone). It uses metal ball and socket of larger diameter, thus reducing the risk of dislocation.

Patello-Femoral Replacement

This is another very rarely performed joint replacement. It can be mostly seen in those individuals who have severe pain on the front of the knee, between the lower part of the thigh bone and the kneecap bone. It is a less invasive surgery with quicker recovery as compared to the total knee replacement.

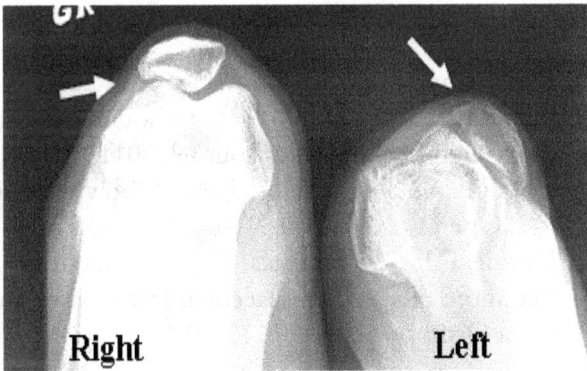

Right   **Left**

Figure 77: Dislocated Patella (knee-cap) compared to normal knee (right)

However, long-term results are not yet available. Most of the studies reveal that 80% to 90% of the patients will have good results, at least for ten years post the patellofemoral replacement.

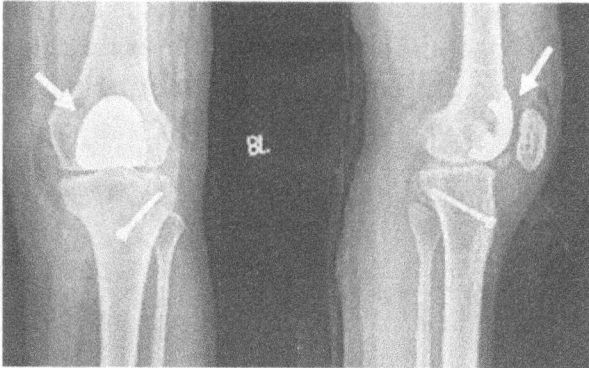

Figure 78: After Patella-femoral replacement (two views of the same knee)

Reference:

1) Sperling JW: Pearls and Tips in Shoulder Arthroplasty. Clin Orthop Surg. 2019 Sep;11(3):258-264.
2) Joaquin Sanchez-Sotelo: Total Shoulder Arthroplasty The Open Orthopaedics Journal, 2011, 5,106-114.
3) Joaquin Sanchez-Sotelo: Total Elbow Arthroplasty, The Open Orthopaedics Journal, 2011, 5, 115-123.
4) Davide Edoardo Bonasia, Federico Dettoni, John E Femino: Total ankle replacement: why, when and how? Iowa Orthop J. 2010;30:119-30.

Case 21: Total Shoulder Replacement

Mr David (name changed), a 60-year-old businessman, had been suffering from shoulder infection since his 20s. Initially, his condition was treated with surgery, and he was put on prolonged antibiotics. However, the infection had damaged the joint cartilage completely, and the situation got worse over the next three decades that followed — his shoulder was worn out severely.

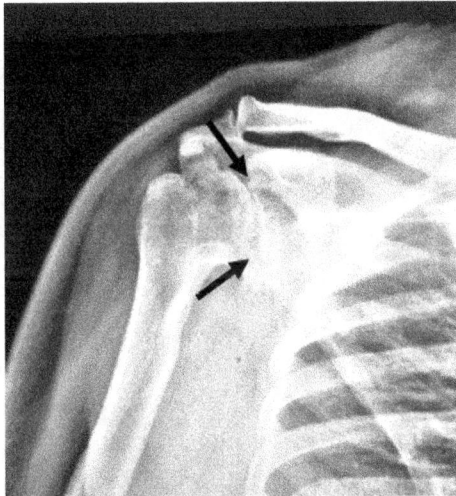

Figure 79: Arthritic shoulder joint with obliteration of joint space

David started facing difficulties in his daily activities like brushing teeth, eating, and even combing his hair. After a course of unsuccessful non-operative treatment and shoulder injection, he finally decided to go for a shoulder replacement.

Interestingly, shoulder replacement is not that commonly performed, unlike knee replacements. So, David was not aware of any patient who had undergone a shoulder replacement to understand the outcomes from a patient's perspective. Thus, he wasn't very sure about the surgery. But the severe pain forced him to do it anyway.

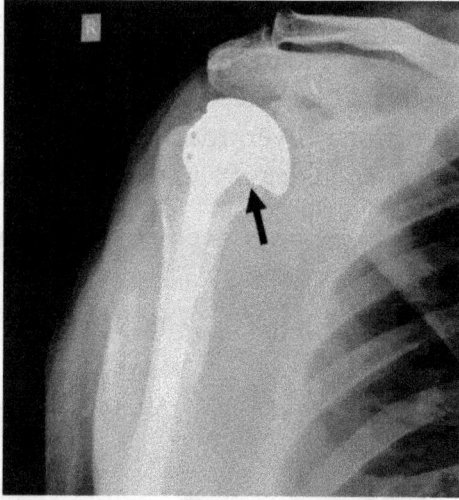

Figure 80: Total shoulder replacement

He underwent a successful total shoulder replacement and was sent back home just two days after surgery. Within six weeks, he was able to return to most of his daily activities; however, over the head activities was something that he could not get back to. He was also advised to avoid heavy manual activities using the operated arm.

David is now extremely happy as he can perform all his daily activities on his own, pain-free.

Case 22: Reverse Shoulder Replacement

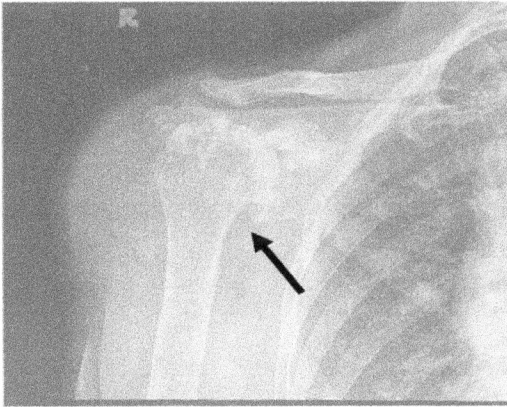

Figure 81: Arthritic Shoulder joint with ball and socket rubbing at each other and the ball migrated upwards

Mrs. Reeta Singh (name changed), a 70-year-old retired telecom officer, had been suffering from shoulder pain for over five years. She recently had to be rushed to the emergency room after experiencing severe pain in the middle of the night. Doctors found out that her shoulder had been dislocated (ball of the joint was moved out of the socket, figure 82).

For momentary relief, the doctors pulled her shoulder back to the original position and gave her a sling.

However, she was in for recurrent episodes of dislocations in the days that followed, and this put Mrs Singh in extreme pain, resulting in frequent visits to the hospital. The X-ray of her shoulder showed severe wear and tear (figure 81), and the MRI scan revealed a complete tear of her shoulder muscles called the 'rotator cuff'. For context, when the rotator cuff is torn, patients develop accelerated wear, and a total shoulder replacement cannot be done in these cases.

Mrs. Singh underwent an operation called reverse shoulder replacement (figure 83), which, by the way, is very popular nowadays. It's been 16 months, and she has shown rapid progress, recovery-wise. She has also been relieved from her nightmares of having further dislocations in the middle of the night.

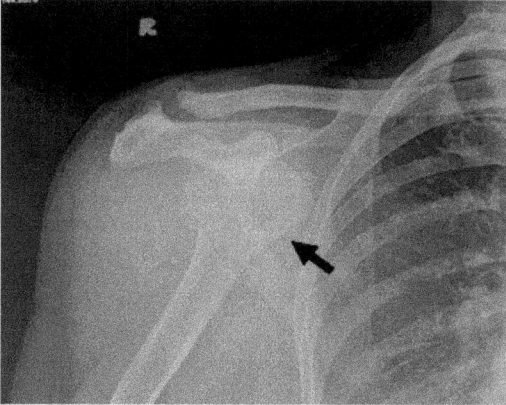

Figure 82: Dislocated ball and socket joint of the shoulder

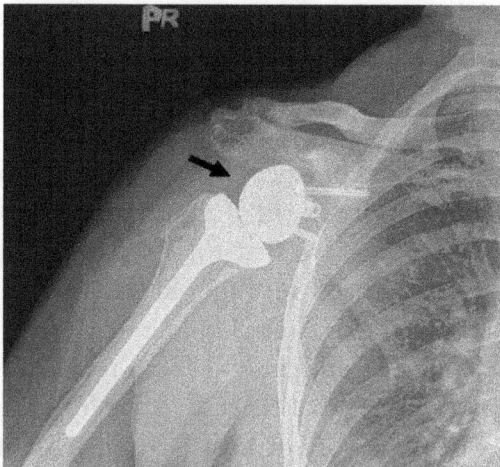

Figure 83: Radiograph showing metal, reverse shoulder prosthesis

Case 23: Total Elbow Replacement

This is another rare joint replacement. Mrs. Vidya (name changed), a 65-year-old lady suffering from multiple joint pains, was on regular rheumatoid medicines for many years. Initially, she had developed a lot of pain in the left big toe, which had affected her walking ability and even caused difficulty in wearing shoes. She had undergone a small surgery and had recovered completely; however, her rheumatoid arthritis had progressively damaged her elbow joint.

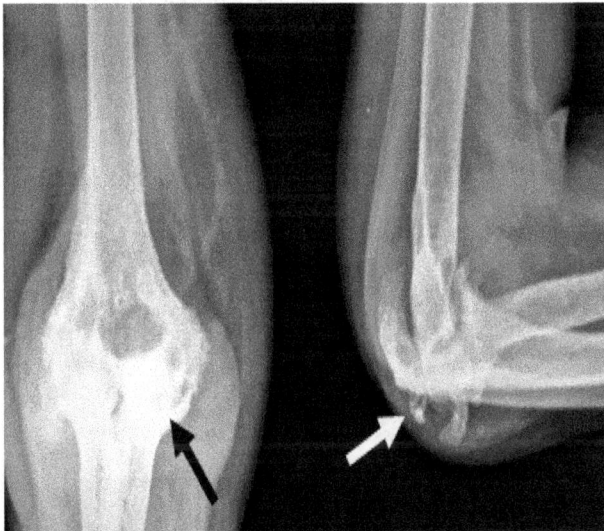

Figure 84: Radiographs of the elbow showing damaged joints

In the next three years, she even developed difficulty in basic daily activities like combing, brushing, and eating. Severe pain was felt in her right elbow, which made her take a lot of pain killers. She was not very keen on getting surgery, and the fact that elbow replacement is rare made her even more sceptical about the surgery.

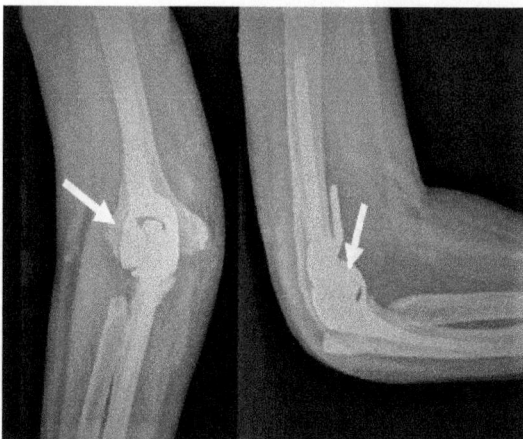

Figure 85: After elbow replacement

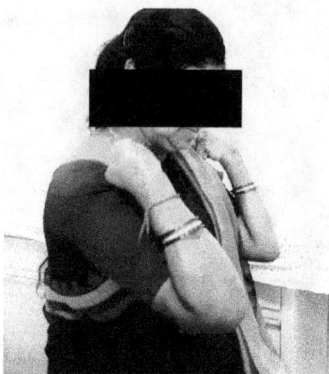

**Figure 86: Ability to
bend completely
after surgery**

**Figure 87:
Ability to
straighten
completely
after surgery**

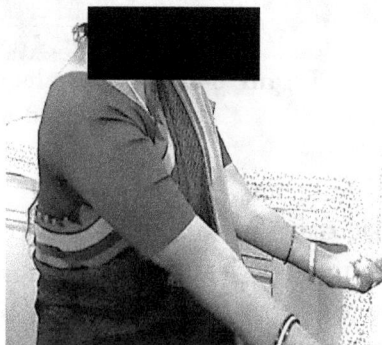

Finally, giving in to her severe pain, she underwent the replacement surgery, and to her own surprise, she recovered within six weeks. She was pain-free and got back to all her daily activities. Seven years since the surgery, Mrs. Vidya is absolutely fine and is going about her daily activities.

DR. NARAYAN HULSE

11
WHICH METAL AND DESIGNS ARE BEST FOR YOU?

Summary:
Even though several methods are used in joint reconstruction, some of them may be outdated, and others may be untested. It is wrong to choose a new implant or metal without scientific evidence, experience in a large number of patients and a long follow up period.

Several designs of joint replacements and a variety of materials have been introduced over the last 70 years. When several options with similar results are available, it isn't easy to objectively compare them, even for doctors. There is no single metal, design, or a company that stands out as many of them have performed equally well. In the end, it all comes to your surgeon's choice, experience and preference, and of course, the requirement of the patient.

The advertisements appearing in print, digital, or any form of media might end up misguiding the patient.

Although the new models in the market claim to be 'high tech,' 'advanced,' and whatnot, sticking with a tried and trusted model is the best way to go about it. Moreover, the efficiency of an implant can be judged only by the scientific community using their different research techniques. Many of these new implants are also driven by marketing forces that can indirectly influence the patient.

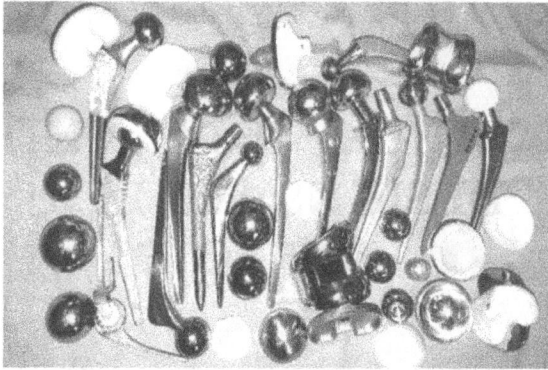

Figure 88: Which one to choose ...!

How Do You Decide?

You must consider the following points.

- **How long has this design been used for?**
The longer, the better. An artificial joint may show catastrophic complications even after many years. Opt for an established knee design that has been used for 10 to 20 years straight.
- **Is it being used in large numbers? It might be an established brand, but is this specific design proven to be successful in a large number of patients?**
Only a prospective study involving a large number of patients can unearth real problems.

- **How good are the long-term results?**

The current standard — Around 90% chances of the implant's survival for at least ten years.

- **What does the National Joint Registries say?**

These are large databases maintained in many countries that have records of patients who have had total joint replacements. National joint registries of the UK, Australia, Sweden, Norway, and Finland have contributed enormous amounts of scientific data to research and understanding of joint replacement surgery.

Results documented in joint registries are the most reliable sources of information regarding the outcomes of the joint replacement surgery.

- **What is the cost of the implant?**

Always remember that the quality of the product has got nothing to do with its price. Most of the newly introduced prostheses are sold for higher rates than the old ones, and this is solely because of the claims that they make which, by the way, might not even be certified.

The established designs, on the other hand, might be cheaper as they are used in a large number of patients for many years.

- **Trust your surgeon.**

An experienced surgeon can help you with the decision-making process as his/her training and experience might be specific to certain prostheses and techniques. Also, the surgeon's experience of using a specific implant is crucial for a successful operation.

Biomaterials for Joints

These materials should be biocompatible, strong to withstand the joint forces' biomechanical forces, and should have excellent wear properties to last longer.

Below listed are the commonly used materials.

Cobalt Chromium Alloy

This alloy is the go-to metal for knee replacements. It is inert, bio-compatible, and the sturdiness provides a suitable moving surface for artificial joints.

However, two metal surfaces coming in contact can produce metal ions, which can reach several parts of the body. But so far, there is no evidence found to prove any harmful effects of these ions.

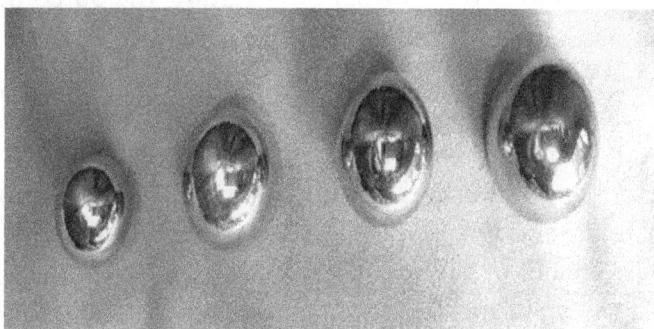

Figure 89: Cobalt chromium metal balls used in hip replacements

In a total knee implant, there will be a polyethylene spacer or an insert in between the two cobalt chrome surfaces. This plastic-like spacer prevents two metal surfaces from rubbing against each other, reducing the number of metal ions being produced in the body.

Nickel, in this alloy, can cause metal allergy in some patients. If a patient has an allergy to metal jewellery, he/she may be at a higher risk of developing an allergy to the implants. This is controversial as skin allergy will not always correlate with the metal implant sitting deep in the joint.

Titanium Alloys

Titanium and its alloys are also one of the commonly used orthopaedic materials. The elasticity of titanium is closest to natural bone, as measured by Young's modulus of elasticity. This alloy also makes a good fit for the plates and nails used in fracture fixations. Titanium, interestingly, has high mechanical strength, excellent corrosion resistance, and biocompatibility with bone.

Titanium and its alloys are preferred in total hip replacements but not so much in total knee implants. It is used in manufacturing the uncemented sockets and stems in the hip, but titanium is not the best candidate for manufacturing joint surfaces due to their poor wear resistance.

Polyethylene

UHMWPE (Ultra-high molecular weight polyethylene) was first introduced in 1962 as the bearing for the Charnley's hip prosthesis. This material is used extensively in other forms even today — The making of a whole socket or the inner liner of the metal socket in the hips and also, inserts or spacers in all the knee replacements.

Polyethylene being a soft material, can easily wear out when used in combination with metal surfaces. Debris of the polyethylene can interact with immune cells of the body and result in lysis of the bone and loosening of the implants. Thus, polyethylene mediated osteolysis and loosening of the joints are the most serious challenges in hip replacement surgeries today. Highly cross-linked polyethylene [XLPE] was developed to address the wear by hardening of polythene. This process involves using either gamma radiation or electron beam radiation to break the covalent bonds.

It is manufactured using cross-linking, heat treatment, and sterilization while making sure of avoiding exposure to air. Recently, some manufacturers have been using Vitamin E, a natural antioxidant, to improve polyethylene's longevity. In laboratory testing, these liners have demonstrated 95-99% less wear than some other highly cross-linked polyethylene liners.

Ceramics

Ceramics are hard materials that are scratch-resistant, wear-resistant, and extremely biocompatible. But on the other hand, they are also brittle and prone to fractures. Hence the hip implants made from the original alumina ceramic have had higher fracture rates.

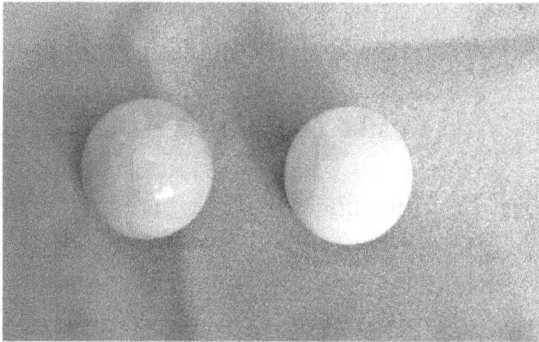

Figure 90: Ceramic balls used in hip replacements

However, the improved manufacturing process reduces the porosity and lowers the granule size of the material, resulting in better toughness and fewer risks of ceramic fractures (delta ceramics).

Zirconia is another ceramic material in combination with alumina that provides increased fracture strength to hip implants. Called Biolox Delta, this combination is very successful at the moment and is used in a large number of patients. This zirconia-toughened alumina (ZTA) has become one of the preferred materials for the hip joint ball, especially in young patients.

Oxinium is a relatively new material produced by heat oxygenation of the zirconium in the presence of air. It forms a layer of black, zirconium oxide on the surface, increases hardness and decreases surface roughness, while also possessing inherently high fracture toughness and fatigue strength because of the metal substrate.

This material is relatively new and needs longer follow-ups. Simulation studies have shown better wear properties, and interestingly, Lewis et al. had compared 50 Co-Cr and 50 Oxinium heads and found the clinical outcome to be equivalent after two years of follow-up.

To add on, Oxinium is also used to produce knee implants, but it is a bit expensive, comparatively. Currently, available research indicates Oxinium based implants did not exhibit lower rates of revision surgeries when compared to Co-Cr implants, across age groups with TKR.

Designs of The Knee Prosthesis

The knee replacement has evolved over the last five decades, and over time, several techniques, materials, and implant designs have been introduced. Some of them are excellent and have changed the orthopaedic practice all over the world with improved outcomes.

However, the point to note here is that some of these innovations have made no significant contribution to the knee replacement procedure and are only pure commercial entities. For example, the uncemented technique of total knee replacement is available but has made no significant difference to the results.

The surgical choice of the implant depends on the complexity of the case, such as major bone loss due to arthritis, previous trauma, or previous surgeries and loss of ligament support.

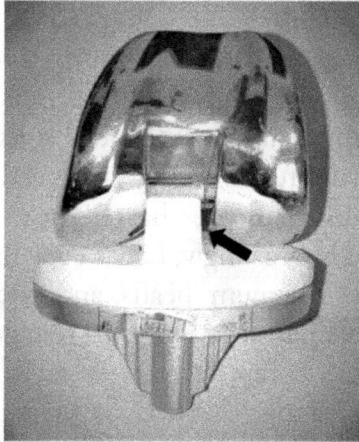

Figure 91: Post and Box (Cam) mechanism of posterior stabilized knees

Cruciate Retaining Total Knees:

This design helps to retain the posterior cruciate ligament, one of the core knee ligaments that provides stability while walking. The theoretical advantages include better roll back and more natural gait, especially while climbing the stairs, bone preservation, and less strain on the metal-bone interface. However, these claims are difficult to establish in clinical studies.

Reported disadvantages include difficulty in balancing the flexion space. In a chronically arthritic knee, posterior cruciate ligament [PCL] may not be functional or may be incompetent, especially in rheumatoid arthritis.

Posterior Stabilized Knee (PS)

Cruciate substituting or posterior stabilized knees have a post-cam mechanism to prevent instability. Here, the posterior cruciate ligament is removed, and the loss of this ligament is substituted in the prosthesis mechanism itself. Currently, this is one of the commonly used designs. Indications for PCL retaining, and cruciate substituting designs are still controversial. Multiple studies have found no significant differences in the function, patient satisfaction, or survivorship between these two designs.

Mobile Bearing Prostheses Vs Fixed Bearing Prosthesis

Mobile-bearing knees were introduced to reduce the stress at the bone-prosthesis interface, and some degree of mobility was incorporated between the polyethylene insert and the tibial component. Potential advantages of mobile bearing knees include lower contact stresses at the articulating surfaces, the rotational motion of the tibial polyethylene during gait, and the self- alignment of the tibial polyethylene compensating for small rotational malalignment of the tibial baseplate during implantation.

Many research studies have failed to establish a clear advantage of one over the other. Fixed bearing total knee replacements continue to be used in the overwhelming majority of the patients in the world.

High Flexion Knee

There is always a demand for higher function and flexibility of artificial knees, depending on the cultural needs of different societies, geographical location, and religious customs.

Remember that the primary goal of a knee replacement is only to provide a durable, painless knee in the elderly. Enabling higher activities like jumping, running and contact sports may not be necessary for this age group. Patients who undergo total knee arthroplasty achieve about 110 to 120 degrees of knee bending on average, which should easily suffice for all the daily activities in elderly patients.

The amount of flexion in the knee depends on multiple factors like preoperative flexion, body weight, and various component designs. The most consistent predictor of postoperative flexion is the range of preoperative flexion.

Several attempts have been made in changing knee prostheses' designs to improve the range of bending of these implants. However, results shown in experimental settings have not been reproduced convincingly in human knees.

Several high-flexion prostheses are now available and have demonstrated variable results. Even though the initial enthusiasm to use these prostheses was partly driven by the commercial interest, high- flexion designs have failed to show statistically significant improvements in knee bending when compared to the standard prosthesis.

Gender-Specific Knee

Surgeons have always observed some disparity between the size and shape of male and female bones. This is the reason gender-specific knees are developed with slightly narrower sizes for women.

Theoretically, these designs fit more accurately and result in less impingement on the surrounding structures.

However, several studies have shown no significant difference between these designs and conventional designs.

Cemented vs Uncemented Knees

Bone cement, which has been used extensively in the knee and hip arthroplasties for about 70 years, has remained the gold standard for fixation of the knee implants. Several attempts have been made so far in developing uncemented knee prostheses but only with little success.

Cementless fixation, on the other hand, has seen a lot of success in total hip arthroplasty, but not so much in total knee replacement. Also, cementless implants are usually made of materials that attract new bone growth.

Constrained, Hinged, Rotating Flatform Knees

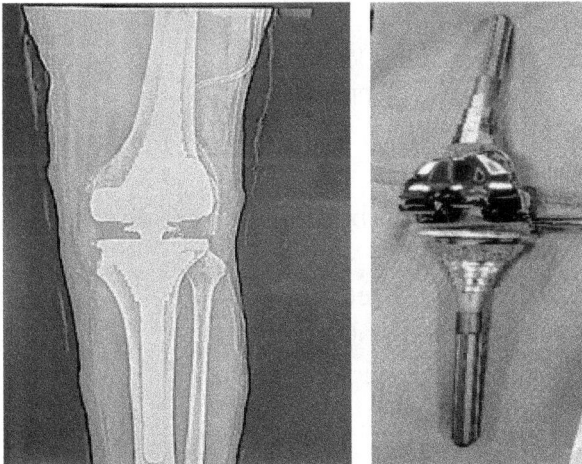

Figure 92: X-ray of a hinged knee replacement and the real prosthesis

These designs are not ideal for primary knee replacements and are used only to salvage failed knee replacements or severely damaged knees in case of arthritic conditions.

These designs are also used in complex and revision scenarios compensating for destroyed ligaments and bone loss.

Designs of Total Hip Replacements

Total hip replacement is one of the best operations available to improve the quality of life. With several modifications and designs, the implants are in use since the 1960s. Given the fact that there is no consensus in the scientific literature regarding the single best hip replacement, each orthopedic surgeon could give you a variety of choices depending on his training and experience. Following are the main types of joint surfaces available

a) Cemented THRs
b) Uncemented THRs
c) Hybrid THRs

And following are bearing surfaces or materials

a) Metal-on-polyethylene,
b) Ceramic-on-polyethylene,
c) Ceramic-on-ceramic,
d) Metal-on-metal

Cemented THR

Cemented total hip replacement is the first significant invention in the history of arthroplasty. In fact, it is also the first successful design developed by Sir John Charnley in the 1960s, which is extensively used even today. It is considered the gold standard in comparison to other models and techniques in the field.

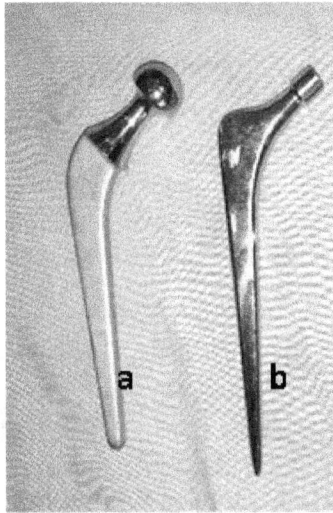

Figure 93: Cemented hips
a) Charnley's type b) Exeter type

In early studies, implant failure after primary THR was attributed to the wear products of cement; it was called "cement disease." However, it is now well known that loosening and failure of the joint replacements were due to polyethylene wear products rather than cement. And this phenomenon is now called "poly disease". At the moment, there is very little evidence to prove that other types of fixations are better than cemented.

Cemented hips are quite popular in Europe compared

to North America. In cemented designs, both socket and stem are fixed inside the bone using bone cement (Poly Methyl Methacrylate); it acts like grout rather than glue.

The advantage of this system is that cement becomes rock-solid in just 10-15 min, and the patients can be fully weight-bearing immediately. Thus, cement also reinforces if the bone is weak and osteoporotic.

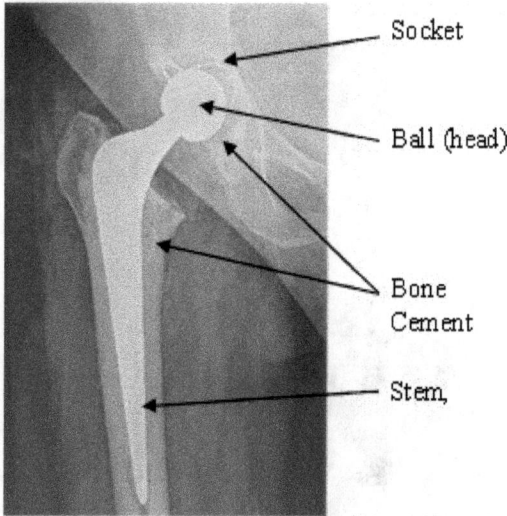

Figure 94: Typical cemented hip replacement

There are mainly two prototypes of cemented hips (figure 93). One is the original Charnley design (Composite beam technique), and the other is the later-developed design by Exeter group in the UK (controlled subsidence), which becomes one of the most successful hips in the history. Additionally, cemented designs are cheaper and have had successful follow-ups in millions of people. The main problem with them, however, is the early failure of the socket, especially in active young patients. Success also depends on the meticulous cementing technique.

Cementless THR:

Uncemented designs are currently the most popular designs of total hip replacements all over the world. While cementing techniques were still being evolved, perceived shortcomings of cement lead to the development of cementless models in North America.

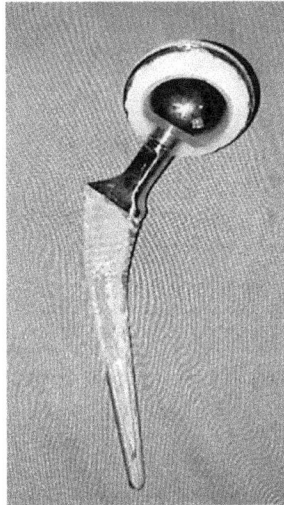

Figure 95: Cementless total hip prototype

Uncemented implants have specialized surfaces to achieve stronger fixation with the bone. Some of these designs have rough surfaces. Currently, most of them have a coating of hydroxyapatite, that allows ingrowth of bone and allows fixation of the prosthesis.

Cementless techniques are easier and quicker. They may be able to preserve some part of the bone in younger patients needing revision later. According to some researcher, it may also be easier to revise these implants if necessary. In the current scientific literature, cementless sockets probably last longer. Now, the superiority of the cemented or cementless variety has remained controversial with no single winner.

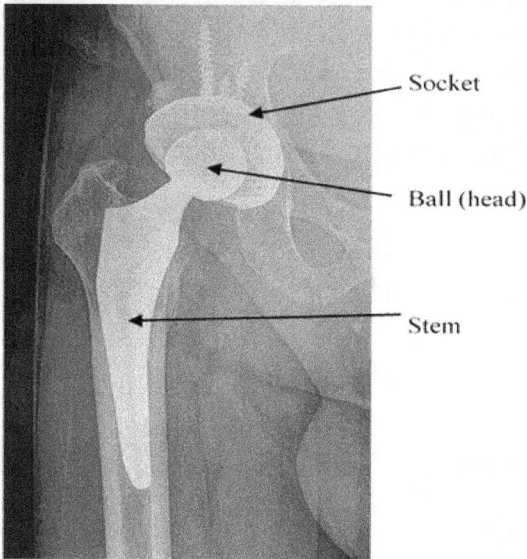

Figure 96: A typical cementless hip prosthesis

Hybrid THR:

Hybrid THR is a technique that has been advocated by some researchers. In this technique, the socket is cementless, whereas the stem is cemented. Some researchers advocate this method for young patients to improve the fixation and thereby the longevity of the artificial socket. There is very little scientific evidence on this technique as the combination is seldom used.

Bearing Surfaces

These are the surfaces on which the hip movement takes place. These materials are used to make the ball and sockets of the hip prosthesis. The structural properties of these materials are crucial because they have to withstand a variety of mechanical forces across the joint. Several designs and combinations of a variety of materials have been tried to find an ideal couple of bearing surfaces, and the below-listed are the commonly used materials:

Metal on Polyethylene

Metal on polyethylene is the most popular combination of bearing surfaces, and for many, it represents the gold standard in total hip arthroplasty. In this design, the acetabular cup is made up of polyethylene, and the ball of the joint is made up of cobalt-chromium alloy. Sir John Charnley originally designed this model and called this combination as low friction arthroplasty. Long term survival of these early implants was good, with 77-81% not needing revision even 25 years after primary THR.

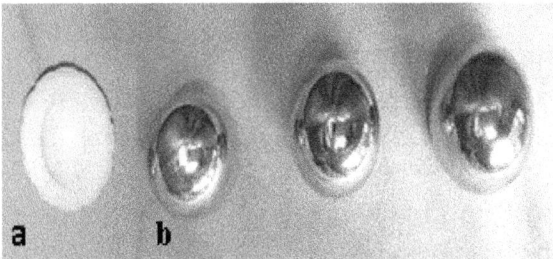

Figure 97: a) Polyethylene socket and b) various sizes of metal balls or heads

Although there was an issue with the polyethylene wear in the earlier designs, it has undergone further development [cross-linking, discussed earlier]. The ultra-highly cross-linked polyethylene (UHXLPE) currently used is harder and has lesser rates of wear.

The main concern of this bearing surface is the wear particles of the polyethylene that can cause osteolysis or a process of dissolving the bone around the prosthesis. As more and more bone substance dissolve, prosthesis becomes loose, and the implant fails.

Osteolysis can also lead to a severe loss of bone, making revision surgeries extremely difficult and less successful. Polyethylene mediated osteolysis is the ultimate cause of failure of most total joint arthroplasties today. To reduce further wear, the toughness of polyethylene has been improved with a variety of techniques.

Metal-on-Polyethylene has been the top bearing surface used by surgeons of many generations since its inception. Several millions of these devices are successfully implanted all over the world. It is also the least expensive bearing. Hence, this bearing combination provides a safe, successful, and cost-effective method for most patients.

Ceramic-on-Ceramic

Ceramic-on-Ceramic is ideal for young patients. It is brittle, tough, scratch-resistant, and has excellent wear properties and biocompatibility. In the hip, ceramic ball (femoral head) can be used in combination with a ceramic socket or a polyethylene socket. In terms of wear reduction, ceramic on ceramic is the best available combination for a hip replacement.

Having been used in hip arthroplasty since the 1980s, ceramic-on-ceramic are also used extensively in dentistry. Additionally, they are the hardest biomaterial with wear rates at about 1000 times less than metal on polyethylene hip replacements.

Historically there are two main problems with ceramic hips. Firstly, they are prone to fractures easily due to their brittleness and the catastrophic complication calls for a revision surgery in the majority of the patients. Secondly, the annoying squeaky noise that arises from the joint. This sound is usually heard only by the patient, causes no pain, and may disappear over time without treatments. Ceramic-on- ceramic is also costlier than any other combinations. However, both these drawbacks have been largely overcome by the newer generation of ceramics and latest techniques.

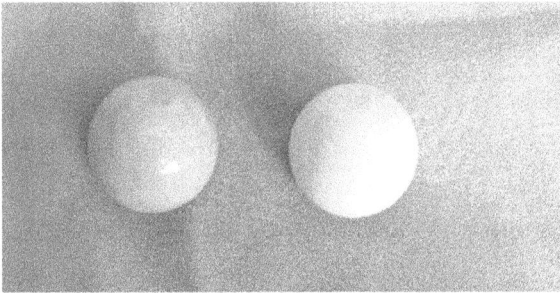

Figure 98: Ceramic balls used in hips

Ceramic-on-Polyethylene

Ceramic ball combined with a polyethylene socket has the advantage of metal on polyethylene and ceramic on ceramic hips. This combination reduces the wear rates significantly compared to the metal on polyethylene hips. Most importantly, the fractures and squeaking associated with the ceramic are also abolished.

The earlier polyethylene cups had higher wear rates, however, the current generation of polyethylene, as discussed earlier, is tough with very low wear rates because of cross-linking.

The ceramic-on-polyethylene combination has wear-rates of about 0.05 millimetres each year, i.e., 50% less than metal-on-polyethylene. The newer, highly cross-linked polyethylene liners, on the other hand, have shown potential wear rates as little as 0.01 millimetres each year.

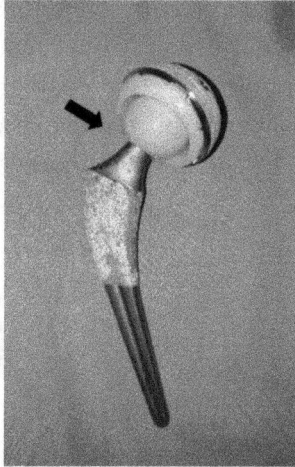

Figure 99: Uncemented hip with Ceramic head

Metal-on-Metal (MoM)

Because of safety reasons and higher failure rates, metal-on-metal implants have become less popular these days. In 2011, the FDA issued a communication regarding metal-on-metal implants, indicating their concerns.

The metal-on-metal implants were in use much before the approval of the FDA in 1999. The metal-on-metal combination allows the largest diameter of heads and sockets compared to any other material; the larger the diameter, the lesser the risks of dislocation. Additionally, as the metal implants are hard and have an ultra-smooth surface, the wear rate is also relatively low. However, there is still the fear of wear products and the microscopic metal ions reaching different body parts via blood; there is no evidence so far to suggest that metal ions can cause any major harmful effects.

Higher rates of failure of these implants may also be because of poor designs and improper implantation techniques rather than the metal-on-metal material themselves.

References

1) Niemeläinen MJ, Mäkelä KT, Robertsson O, et all :The effect of fixation type on the survivorship of contemporary total knee arthroplasty in patients younger than 65 years of age: a register-based study of 115,177 knees in the Nordic Arthroplasty Register Association (NARA) 2000-2016. Acta Orthop. 2020 Apr;91(2):184-190.

2) Zagra L: Advances in hip arthroplasty surgery: what is justified? EFORT Open Rev. 2017 May 11;2(5):171-178.

3) Chang Yong Hu, Taek-Rim Yoon: Recent updates for biomaterials used in total hip arthroplasty: Biomater Res. 2018 Dec 5;22:33.

4) Vertullo CJ, Lewis PL, Graves S, Kelly L, Lorimer M, Myers P: Twelve-Year Outcomes of an Oxinium Total Knee Replacement Compared with the Same Cobalt-Chromium Design: An Analysis of 17,577 Prostheses from the Australian Orthopaedic Association. National Joint Replacement Registry. J Bone Joint Surg Am. 2017 Feb 15;99(4):275-283.

Case 24: This Doctor Conducted a Caesarean Delivery, Four Weeks After Her Both Knee Replacements!

Dr Shobha [name changed] is a 60-year-old famous gynaecologist and renowned professor of obstetrics and gynaecology. She had been suffering from severe pain in both her knees for over ten years.

When it comes to medical issues, doctors are no different. She consulted several orthopaedic surgeons and underwent several nonsurgical treatments — She took a long time to consider joint replacement. In the end, when she could not bear the pain anymore, she finally decided to undergo a total knee replacement.

She was a typical osteoarthritic patient with mild bowing of her legs. She was also slightly overweight. Interestingly, Dr Shoba comes from a family of doctors. Her son, a physician himself, had read in detail about the knee replacement surgery. One of the issues that bothered them was the type and the material of the implant that was to be used.

They were aware of cobalt-chromium alloys, titanium and oxonium alloys. Since they were all doctors, it was not difficult for them to understand the importance of long-term follow up of medical devices and their safety record. Everything with glaring publicity and latest brand need not be the best!

She underwent both knee replacements using standard implants made from cobalt-chromium alloy. She recovered well without any complications. She was very co-operative, enthusiastic, and prompt in her rehabilitation and physiotherapy.

Dr Shobha had a lot of patients rooting for her; she was their favourite. During her recovery phase, one of her patients requested her to conduct the delivery of their first child. She took up the challenge and performed a C-section, and this was just in four weeks of her knee replacements.

To everybody's delight, the new-born baby, first-time mom and their beloved doctor with a pair of new knees were all fine, and they all celebrated together!

Case 25: Her Metal-on-Metal Hip Resurfacing Did Not Work for Long

Fifty-eight-year-old Ashia (name changed) had undergone a hip surgery five years ago. She had suffered a condition called avascular necrosis of the hip, and in this condition, the blood supply to the hip joint (femoral head) is blocked for a variety of reasons. The exact cause of this problem remains unknown in most of the patients.

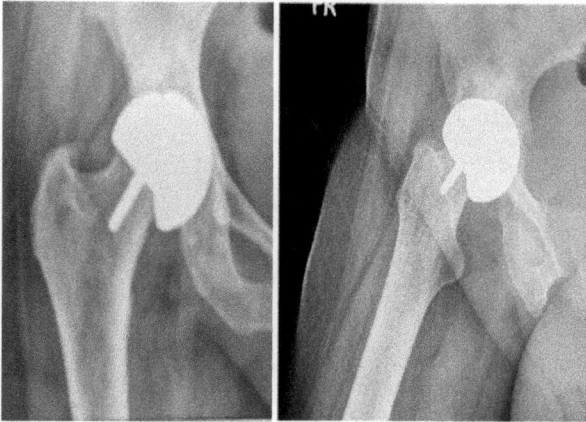

Figure 100: Slipped socket of the hip resurfacing implant

Her son being a doctor himself, wanted to choose the best available hip replacement for his mother. After several consultations and research on the types of prosthesis available, she underwent a metal-on-metal type of hip resurfacing, as it was the 'latest' technology then.

In the late 1990s and the decade that followed, there was a trend to use this prosthesis as an alternative to traditional hip replacement in young people, all over the world. These 'latest' methods claimed to be superior and to last longer than traditional replacements.

However, a high percentage of failures were seen in their usage, and the manufacturers ended up scraping their prosthesis. Even the FDA disapproved of this product eventually.

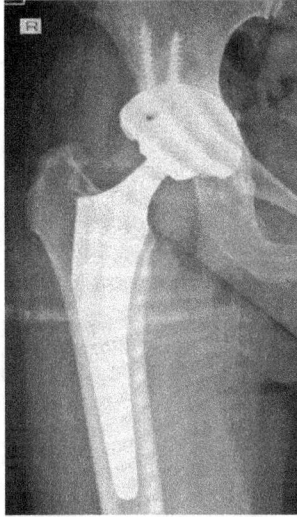

Figure 101: After a revision hip replacement

Mrs. Ashia was in a pickle. The surgery gave her no comfort whatsoever. In fact, from the day of her surgery, the pain intensified. She continued to limp and experienced severe pain in her hip. An X-ray that was taken at this stage revealed a completely failed hip resurfacing. Mrs. Ashia then underwent the right revision hip replacement and recovered well.

The moral of the story is not to go behind the 'latest' and 'fancy' implants. Long term scientific research and follow up showing good results should be the top priority when considering joint replacements.

Case 26: Her Bone Was Worn Out and Weakened So Much That It Broke Without Any Injury!

Mrs. Maya (name changed), a 65-year-old lady, had always been sceptical of modern medicine. Even though she was suffering from severe knee pain and had been experiencing difficulty in walking for over ten years, she refused to even consider knee replacement. She was also suffering from diabetes and hypertension.

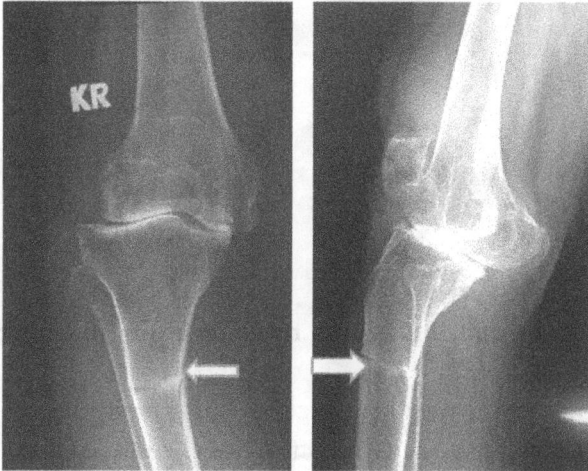

Figure 102: Spontaneous Fracture of the leg bone called stress fracture

Maya was able to walk inside the house with the help of a walker, but she suddenly experienced the onset of severe pain in her right leg one day. The X-ray report showed a small crack in the leg bone just below the knee joint; this is called "stress fracture" (figure 102). This fracture had occurred without any fall or significant trauma. These spontaneous or low energy fractures occur in conditions like 'osteomalacia' and 'osteoporosis'.

Generally, for the bones to remain strong and healthy,

walking is essential along with the intake of adequate quantities of calcium and vitamin D. Patients who have severe arthritis are usually confined to their homes without any sunlight exposure for many years. As sunlight is the primary source of vitamin D, they might end up suffering from osteomalacia and immobility induced osteoporosis.

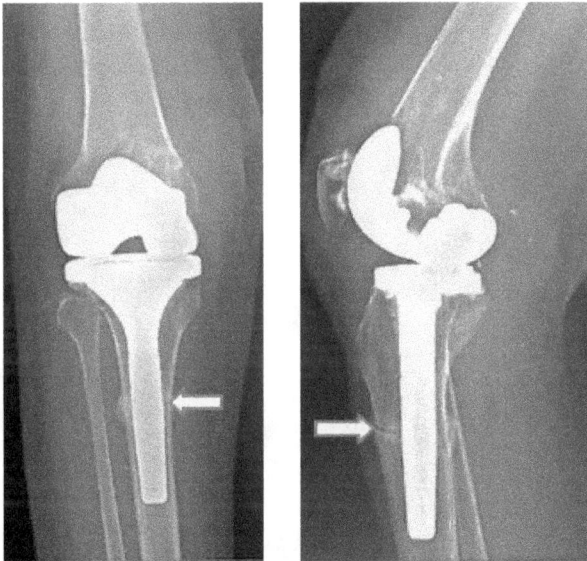

Figure 103: Knee replacement with a stem is used to fix the stress fracture

As someone who believed in alternative therapies like Ayurveda, homoeopathy, and other traditional methods, Maya stayed far away from surgeries. However, she had to finally give in, as her mobility and general health started deteriorating over a period of time. This condition also affected her general health, bone quality, blood pressure and sugar levels.

After a marathon session of counselling, she agreed to undergo the replacement surgery. Because of the stress fracture, Maya had to deal with a more complicated knee replacement. A knee implant with an additional stem was used to fix the fracture simultaneously (figure 103), and the fracture healed in 12 weeks. Finally, she got back to her normal life, relieved of her chronic pain and enjoyed her newly restored mobility.

Case 27: This High Court Lawyer Had One Last Hope!

Mr. Prasad (name changed), a successful high court lawyer in his 50s, had been suffering from an autoimmune neurological disease for over three years. This illness was treated with several medicines by many specialists. The steroid was one of the medications used to suppress the inflammation.

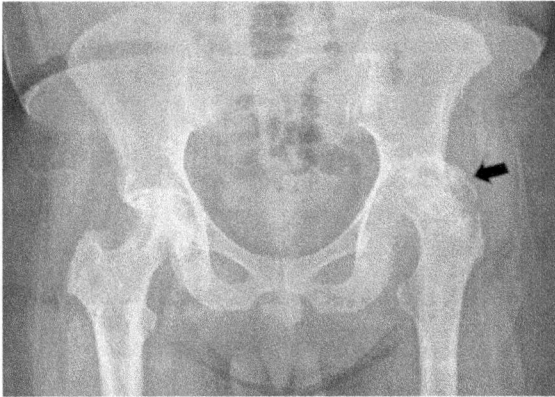

Figure 104: Ball of the hip migrated up into the damaged socket

Steroids can damage the hip joint by blocking the blood supply called avascular necrosis of the hip. Steroids can also suppress the body's immunity against infections. As a result of consuming steroid as a medication, Mr. Prasad ended up with an infection in his hip. An operation was performed, and the infection was taken care of.

By the time he approached me, he was experiencing severe pain in his hip and was emotionally disturbed. His X-ray report revealed extensively damaged hips; both the socket and ball of the hip were completely damaged. Additionally, there was a suspicion of the persisting infection.

He underwent all the medical assessments, and we reasonably ruled out any infection in the hip. All these complications and the fact that his socket was extensively worn out made the surgery a highly complicated procedure. Because the socket was badly damaged and widened, a normal-sized artificial cup could not be inserted. I had to reconstruct the socket using the bone graft. This bone graft was taken from the upper part of his thigh bone, which is normally removed during hip replacement.

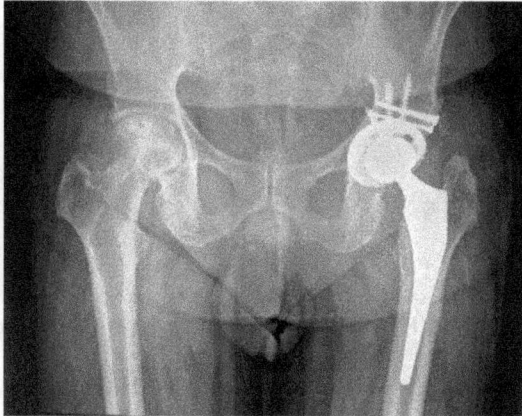

Figure 105: Hip replacement: Height restored to normal. Both sockets are at the same level

He underwent the replacement surgery while being aware of all the complications. He trusted us, so the surgery had to be a success no matter what. And as it turned out, the surgery was indeed a success. He was doing great when I saw him last. The bone graft had healed completely, and he was walking like a normal person without limping or experiencing any pain. In fact, he had already resumed his court proceedings!

12
COMPLICATIONS AND PREVENTION

All medical and surgical procedures are associated with some degree of complications and risks, and joint replacements are no different. Surgical replacement techniques of the knee and hip joints are, in fact, among the most successful and cost-effective interventions in modern medicine. But this is not without risk or complications.

These medical complications can occur after all types of joint replacements, including knee, hip, shoulder etc. However, some risk is specific to the type of joint replacements such as dislocations in hip joints.

Also, it is essential to understand all the possible outcomes before consenting for surgery. Doctors and nurses should also emphasize that adverse events can be associated with medical treatments and surgical procedures, despite taking all necessary precautions and care.

The following list, although not exclusive, includes the commonly occurring complications and their prevention.

If a joint replacement fails due to any of the reasons below, further reconstruction is possible, which is discussed in the next chapter.

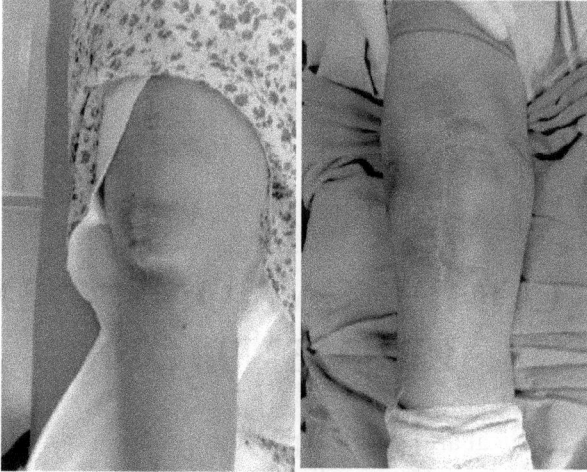

Figure 106: Infection after knee replacements – pus collection and a non-healing wound

Infection

Infection is a condition when microorganisms such as bacteria invade your replaced joints and cause a host of biological damage. This is evidenced by the formation of pus, swelling, fever, not healing wounds, increased pain, and restriction of movements.

Infection after a joint replacement occurs in about 0.5 to 3% of the cases. In a modern hospital, the rate of infection of about 1% or less is an acceptable standard.

Infection control protocols have improved tremendously in the last 70 years. Some of the preventive measures in use are antibiotics (two or three doses only), modern ultra-clean operation theatres, aseptic surgical techniques, laminar flow operation theatres to control the air quality, antibiotic-impregnated bone cement, and body exhaust surgical suites.

Some patients suffering from uncontrolled diseases like diabetes and other vascular diseases, such as reduced blood supply, local trauma with compromised skin, and previous operations with existing metal fixations are at an increased risk of these infections.

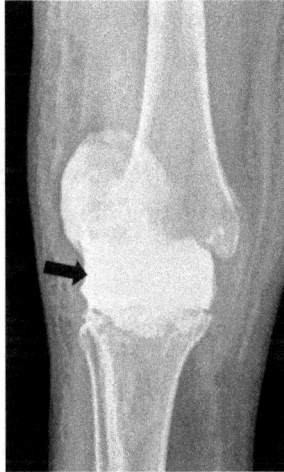

Figure 107: Antibiotic spacer(arrow)that was placed after removing infected joint

Unlike our body parts and organs, infection around metal prosthesis is difficult to control. This is because bacteria form a layer of protein over the metal surface and settle comfortably under this layer. This layer is formed in about three weeks after the onset of infection, making it very difficult to control thereafter.

To diagnose the infection, other than looking at your replaced joint, surgeons may do an X-ray to check for loosening of the implants, conduct a blood test to see increasing parameters like ESR and CRP or remove the fluid from the joint and send it for testing in a laboratory.

If an infection is detected before the bacteria settle, say in about three weeks, an operation called debridement and liner exchange is performed. In this procedure, the knee is cleaned with lots of lavages, and any easily detachable parts are removed and replaced with a new one.

This procedure has a success rate of about 80%. However, this procedure is of no use if the infection is established over three weeks. In this case, a two-staged surgery might be recommended. Following this, all the implants are removed, and an antibiotic mixed cement is placed inside the joint as a spacer (figure 107).

This is then followed by antibiotic therapy for more than a month. Usually, after six to eight weeks, if the infection is fully controlled, a new joint replacement is re-implanted.

Deep Vein Thrombosis (DVT) And Pulmonary Embolism (PE)

The formation of blood clots in the leg veins is common after joint replacement surgeries. The incidence of this complication is higher after total hip replacements than in a knee replacement. These clots usually get dissolved by themselves and do not really cause any problem to the majority of patients.

However, in a small number of patients, these blood clots can dislodge and propagate to other parts of the body. When these clots reach the chest and block the vital blood supply to the lungs, they can be fatal; they may also propagate to heart and rarely, even the brain. This phenomenon is called an embolism, and it can be fatal in about 0.001% of the patients.

Even though pulmonary embolism is rare, it is a severe complication. Therefore, routine DVT prophylaxis is recommended for all the patients undergoing total knee and hip replacements. To prevent several strategies are followed.

• You should stop hormone tablets such as oestrogen or progesterone at least six weeks before surgery.

• All these patients get blood thinners called anticoagulants after the surgery. Some of them are pills, and some are injections. It is important to take these medications regularly as per your surgeon's advice.

• Early mobilization after a joint replacement is essential. Early walking, physiotherapy and exercises prevent stagnation of blood-flow inside the calf muscle.

• You should exercise your ankle once in every half hour when you are awake. These exercises will pump the blood upwards. Hence the name 'ankle pump exercise'.

• You may be advised to wear special stockings called TEDS (Thrombo-Embolic Deterrent Stockings).

• Foot and calf pump machines are available. This can be used all day, especially in those patients who cannot take blood-thinning medications.

• Some patients who are at serious risk of developing a pulmonary embolism or patients who have an existing clot may need a filter placed in the large vessels of the chest (inferior vena cava) to prevent the clots from reaching the lungs.

A combination of practices mentioned above should be followed routinely. For better results, you may need some of these modalities for six to twelve weeks.

Dislocation:

Dislocation is one of the common complications after hip replacements. Here, the ball of the joint comes out of the socket leading to severe pain and inability to walk. This complication can happen in about three per cent of the patients; however, some conditions like hip fractures needing hip replacements may have a higher risk of dislocations of up to 10%. Hip dislocation is more common in patients with muscle weakness, neurological diseases, repeated surgeries, and uncooperative patients who fail to take the right precautions.

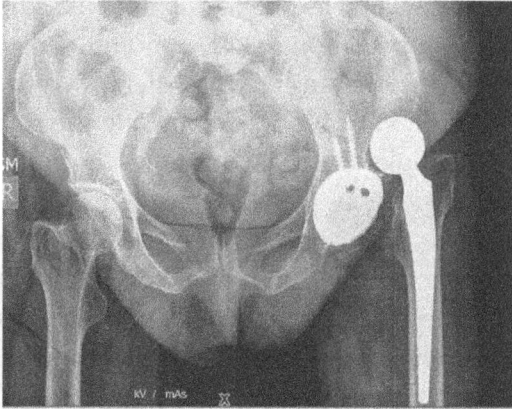

Figure 108: Dislocated total hip replacement

During the surgery, several tests are conducted on the hip to make sure there are no dislocations. If the hip dislocates by any chance, then adjustments are made in the size and orientation of the implants to make it stable. However, if the total hip replacement is dislocated, then hospitalization is the only option.

A closed reduction or manipulation of your hip back to its position is attempted first. This will be done under the influence of some type of anaesthesia. If the hip fails to go back to its position (this is a rare case), you may need open surgery to relocate the hip. Knee replacements can also dislocate, very rarely. These complications are usually due to injuries or ligament imbalances.

Instability

Instability after total knee replacement can be frustrating as the knee is not strong enough to handle normal daily activities. Pain, buckling, difficulty in climbing stairs, or recurrent swellings might be symptoms of instability.

Instability may require revision surgeries, which accounts for about 10-20% of revisions after total knee replacements. It can be seen in about one to two per cent of patients after knee replacements. Late loosening of the implants in the knee, stretching of the ligaments in some diseases such as SLE, or trauma to knee ligaments are some of the causes of instability.

Treatments to this condition also depend on the cause and severity. Minor instability could be managed with bracing and physiotherapy, whereas major instability may need revision surgery.

Vascular Injury

During a surgical procedure, there is a small risk of accidentally damaging the blood vessels around the surgical site. For instance, there are chances of the popliteal artery being injured while cutting the bones with a surgical saw and other surgical steps, during a knee replacement. In these cases, the injury will need to be recognized immediately and repaired by vascular surgeons.

Nerve Palsy

Similarly, during hip and knee replacements, the nerves around the joint can also get damaged. Although it is possible in both cases, it is more frequently seen after hip replacements. This problem usually presents as post-operative 'foot drop' wherein, the patient will find it very difficult to lift the affected foot upwards.

Additionally, patients with complex joint conditions are more prone to nerve damage. Foot-drop is seen more frequently after correction of severe knock-knee, revision knee replacements, congenital dislocations of the hip needing leg- lengthening, and revision hip replacements.

Although most of these injuries recover without any active treatments, it may take a long time, even up to 18 months in some cases.

Initial treatment includes splinting and physical therapy; if the condition gets out of hand, then the patients may require surgical correction.

Wound Complications

Delayed wound healing and sub-optimal healing may be seen rarely in immunocompromised patients after the correction of complex deformities - this may be due to the presence of unhealthy skin or old scars.

Stiffness

Stiffness is another rare complication that comes about after a knee replacement. Your knee replacement is considered stiff if you fail to reach a flexion of about 90 degrees six weeks post-surgery.

This condition may occur in those patients with severe stiff knee even before surgery, along with other conditions like obesity, severe deformities, swollen legs due to other pre-existing medical conditions, and inadequate physiotherapy. Some of these patients may need manipulation under anaesthesia at six weeks and even revision surgeries, in rare cases.

Fractures

Fractures occurring around the components of the joint replacements are called periprosthetic fractures. These fractures are rare, but once they occur, surgery might be inevitable. The Swedish joint registry had revealed in 2000 that the number of periprosthetic fractures had increased from 0.045% in 1975 to 0.13%.

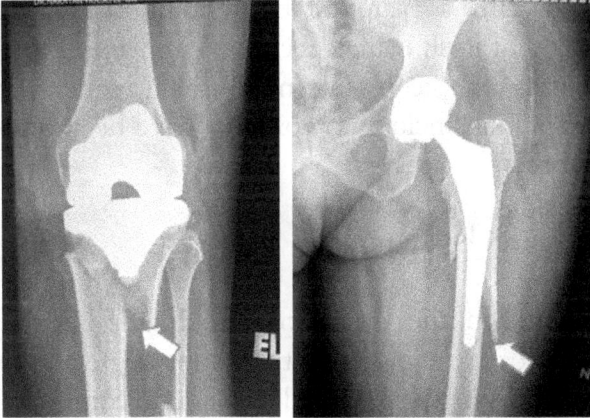

Figure 109: Fractures just below knee and hip replacements

Patients with certain pre-medical conditions are at higher risk of periprosthetic fracture; weak bones and a fall is the most common cause of these fractures.

Some of the other common conditions that might lead to fractures are osteoporosis (week bone with low calcium), osteolysis (progressive local bone loss due to orthopaedic implants), tumours, and weakened implants (fatigue fractures of the implants).

In present times, fractures around the joint replacements are increasing day by day. A number of factors contribute to this — Increasing number of joints operated, increasing age of the patients, increasing revision joint replacements, a growing number of total joint replacements involving joints different from both hip and knee, shoulder and elbow, and also, the popularity of uncemented prosthesis.

Many of these patients require further surgery, and this often gets challenging because of their old age and other pre-conditions that they might be suffering from.

This problem is usually treated either by fixing the fracture with a plate or by redoing the entire joint replacement itself using specialized implants. However, it is crucial to keep in mind that higher rates of complications, including mortality, have been reported in these circumstances.

Change in Leg Length

Change in the length of legs might be a possible outcome of hip replacement; a minor degree of variation in the length of the operated leg is quite common.

A majority of the patients face no functional limitations, but many may be worried about their cosmetic appearances. Significant variations can lead to limping and rarely issues like backache after many years.

However, this discrepancy will be less than 0.5-1cm in majority and can be easily adapted by the body without much discomfort.

Take a look at the following points to know more about this change in length.

• Slight lengthening is more common than shortening.

• While checking the leg length, your pelvis, and both hips should be placed in an identical position; any tilt in the pelvis could lead to an error in the measurement. So, don't try to check it yourself and ask for help!

• If you are limping, it need not be because of shortening only. Limping is common during the first three to four months after the surgery because of pain, stiffness, and muscle weakness.

• During the first week after the operation, your leg always feels longer because of how you tilt your hip and pelvis to relieve the surgical pain.

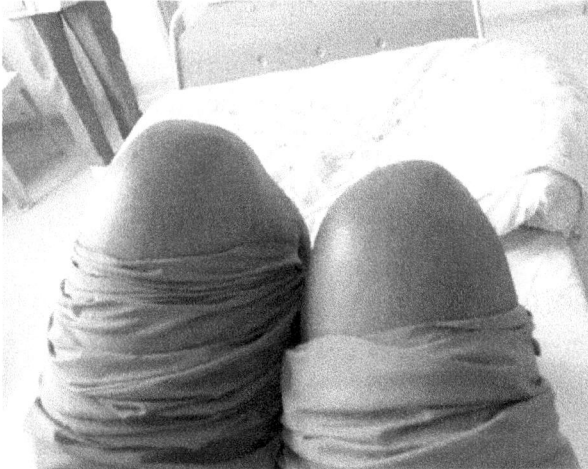

Figure 110: Short right thigh, before hip replacement

• Your surgeon may have to keep the leg a little shorter in case you have a long-term hip problem. If your surgeon attempts to make your hip longer than four centimeters, nerves around the hip may get severely stretched, and this could lead to permanent nerve damage, ultimately resulting in foot-drop. In this situation, functioning hip with intact nerves is a better choice than trying to equalize the length, which may give you a permanent disability.

• Minor shortening can easily be treated with a small shoe raise. Even by the most experienced hands, equalizing the leg length in certain patients with complex hip diseases may not be possible.

• In some cases, surgeon may have to make the leg a little longer; this situation happens if your hip and tissues are too loose. The tightening of the tissues by placing a longer implant might be necessary. If not tightened, the artificial hip may become unstable and dislocate after surgery.

• Surgeon may also keep the leg a little longer if you are expected to have the other hip replaced soon as well. In fact, it is easier to make the hip a little longer than shorter while performing the other hip replacement on a later date.

Implant Loosening

This phenomenon of loosening heralds the ultimate failure of the joint replacements. The implant may loosen if it is not strongly fixed due to any reason during the surgery. This is also quite common if you exert any type of mechanical force or meet with an accident.

However, the usual mechanism is a gradual immune-mediated loss of the bone around the implant called lysis. Because of this, the supporting bone becomes weaker and fails to support the implant.

Loose implants can cause severe pain and hinder your mobility. Thus, most of the patients need revision joint replacements. In the last seventy years, use of advanced materials and techniques have reduced the rate of implant loosening and most of the implants last over two decades in more than 90% of patients.

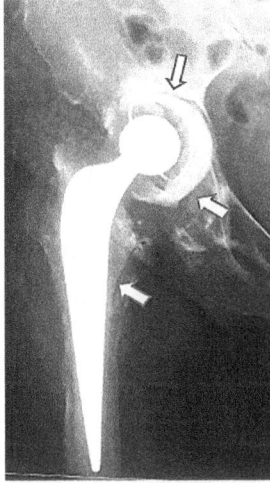

Figure 111: Hip Implant loosening: X rays showing a gap between the bone and implant

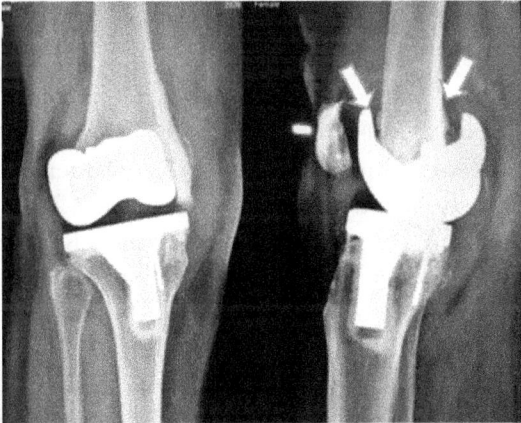

Figure 112: Knee implant loosening: X rays showing the gap between the bone and implant

Other Complications:

• Regional pain syndrome, patellar complications, anterior knee pain, anesthesia complications, mortality, allergies, are possible but pretty rare.

- Mortality rate is about 0.4% in 90 days after the joint replacement. This could be because of a variety of medical complications.
- Re-operations: 3.8% of patients will undergo another surgery to improve the knee pain within four years. These are the surgeries only to deal with some of the complications of the knee replacements.
- Persistent pain: In a study, 5.6% of patients have worse Patient- Reported Outcome Measures (PROM) six months post- surgery, and a Knee Society Score (KSS) of less than 70.18.

These are rare but can be because of unexplained knee pain in some patients. These patients' medical examinations and tests may not reveal any obvious abnormalities.

References:

1) Narayan Hulse: Total knee replacement in arthritis - Current Concepts. Chapter 9. Frontiers in Arthritis, Ashish Anand (ed). 2017, Vol 1, 105-127.

2) Narayan Hulse, Himanshu Sharma, Rana B: Role of vena cava filters in high risk trauma and elective orthopaedic procedures, Current Orthopaedics, 2007, Jan 21(1):72-78.

3) Telissi N, Kakwani R, Narayan Hulse: Autologous blood transfusion following Total Knee arthroplasty, Is it always necessary? Int Orthop. 2006 Oct;30(5):412-4.

4) Gillespie W. Murray D. Gregg P.J. Warwick D: Risks and benefits of prophylaxis against venous thromboembolism in orthopaedic surgery. J Bone Joint Surg Br. 2000; 82: 475-479.

Case 28: He Found His Surgeon While Doing a Literature Search About His Complicated Hips!

Mr Krishnamurthy (name changed), a 65-year-old, had been suffering from damaged hips for over 30 years. Having had multiple failed hip surgeries, he was scared to undergo any further surgery — These failed surgeries had caused infections which resulted in complications like pulmonary embolism.

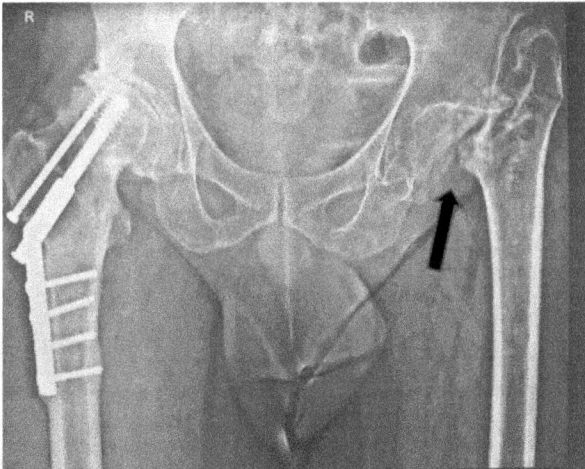

Figure 113: Severely affected right hip after fixation, and a false hip on the right (arrow)

His ordeal started in his thirties when he sustained a road traffic accident and broke his right hip. His hip was operated and fixed with a plate and screw. The fracture healed, and he was able to walk, although he did feel slight discomfort. In fact, he ended up limping for ten years. Eventually, the blood supply to both his hips also started to diminish — This condition is called avascular necrosis of the hip.

He had to undergo another surgery, a hip replacement

in his left hip. It was complicated as there was a severe infection in that area. The infection could not be controlled even after multiple surgeries. His hip replacement implant was then removed, and he was left with a false hip. He later developed a severe pulmonary embolism and needed lifelong blood thinners. After a prolonged period of pain and rehabilitation, he could finally walk with two crutches and manage his basic daily activities on his own.

However, his hips started deteriorating slowly, and he could not bear the pain any longer. He was in his sixties by this time. But, as I mentioned earlier, because of his failed earlier surgeries and complications like pulmonary embolism, he was frightened to undergo any further surgeries.

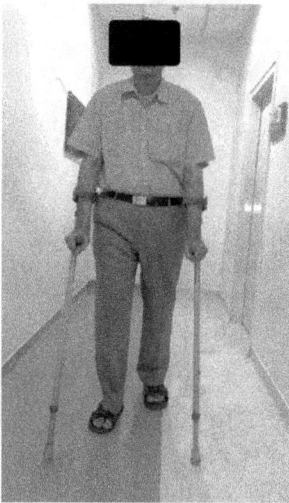

Figure 114: He could walk only with the help of two crutches

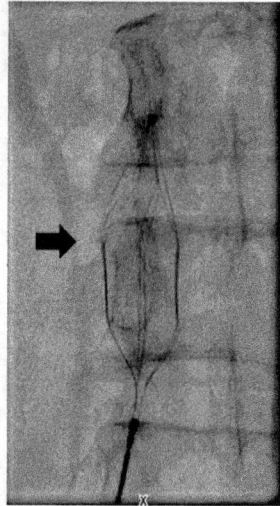

Figure 115: Bird nest type of a filter to prevent clots reaching his heart

So, he started reading up and researching from all the sources available to understand how one could prevent further pulmonary embolism after joint replacements. This is when he came across one of the articles written by me that talked about placing a device in the veins to filter the blood clots (Narayan Hulse et al.: Role of vena cava filters in high-risk trauma and elective orthopaedic procedures, Current Orthopedics, 2007, Jan 21(1):72-78). Influenced by this article, he reached out to me and told me about all the sufferings he was going through.

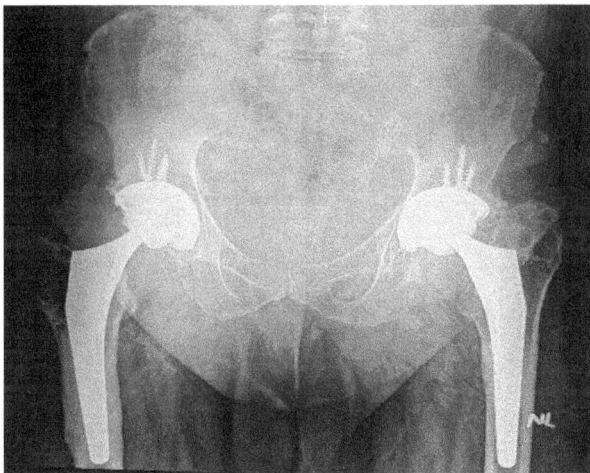

Figure 116: After replacement of his both hips

His hips were severely damaged, and they needed major reconstruction. Because of his previous history of blood clots, he was indeed a high-risk patient. After a great deal of counselling and planning, he was admitted. His blood thinner pills were stopped a week before the surgery to reduce surgical bleeding. A senior cardiologist placed a filter in his veins (Venacaval Filter). Both hip replacements were done in a staged manner at an interval of one week. He recovered well, and the filter was removed after six weeks.

Eight years since his complex hip replacements, he is happy. He walks independently and goes out for evening walks, for about 2 kilometres every day. He even plays with his grandchildren in the park. He tells me that he is forever thankful for his discovery of that article written by me on Venacaval filters!

Case 29: This 90-Year-Old Broke His Hip Replacement While His Surgeon Was Away!

Mr. Wilson (name changed), a 90-year-old man, managed to get by his daily activities using a walking stick. A few years ago, he had sustained a hip fracture, which was treated surgically using a Hemi hip replacement.

Things were fine post-surgery until he slipped and fell again in the washroom. He experienced severe pain in his hip and was unable to walk. He was rushed to the emergency room of the same hospital where his previous replacement surgery was done. Unfortunately, his surgeon was away in a conference for three consecutive days, and so were many other senior surgeons, including me.

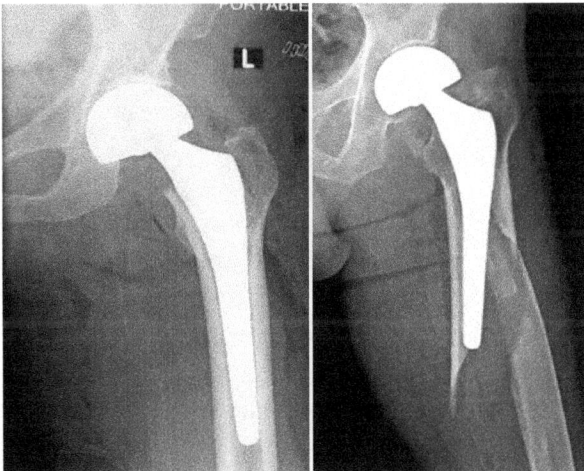

Figure 117: Before and after he sustained a fracture around the hip replacement

Mr. Wilson finally reached our hospital, and I operated on him upon my return after two days. This was the most challenging fracture to operate on as he was a very fragile patient.

This fracture had to be treated by removing the old hip replacement and then fixing the fracture simultaneously using a special hip replacement with a longer stem. There was no other sensible option.

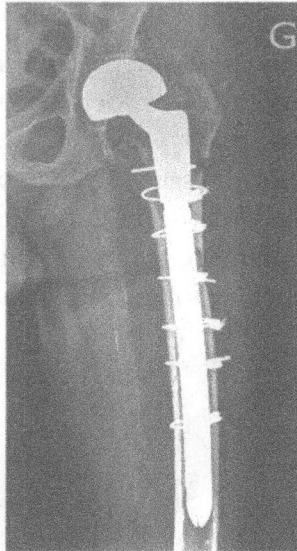

Figure 118: Fracture is fixed using a long- stemmed hip replacement and cables

After the surgery, he was monitored in the intensive care unit. He was moved around on a wheelchair. In about six weeks, he started walking with the help of a walker. He showed rapid progress and began performing his daily activities all by himself.

Mr. Wilson was doing great for over three years of post-surgery, but he came back after suffering another fall. This time, he had broken a shoulder bone, but that was corrected without any operation.

13
EXERCISES AFTER SURGERY

Exercises after knee replacements should be continued even after going home. These exercises should be done three to four times a day, spanning several months. Most of them are simple and can be performed by the patients without any help. Besides exercising, patients should also walk regularly, which should be progressed according to their individual capacity.

Knees take a longer time to rehabilitate than hips. Many patients might take up to eight-twelve weeks. That said, some patients assume that a therapist's guidance is required for over three months, and vigorous physiotherapy must be practised despite the pain — This is a misconception.

Most of the patients can do these exercises without supervision, and patients should never try to exceed their limits. If the patient pushes himself/herself beyond their limits, the increasing pain may inhibit mobility, cause muscle spam, and the patient's morale might go down. These things might make the rehabilitation process exceedingly difficult, painful, and slow.

It is also quite natural to feel some pain and soreness in the muscle post work-out. Although one might be tempted to consume pain-killers, please refrain from excessive usage; they have their own side effects. Ice-packing around the knee helps in reducing pain and swelling, to some extent. If it's too much, you can always stop the exercises for a day or two and resume once you are ready. It is best always to start slow and gradually increase your activity level.

General Exercises for Both Hip and Knee

To prevent Deep Vein Thrombosis [DVT], a condition caused by blood clots in veins located deep inside your legs, ankle pump exercises are a must. For this exercise, move your ankle several times, as shown in figures 119 and 120. These exercises should be done until the swellings are completely subsided, and you are fully mobile.

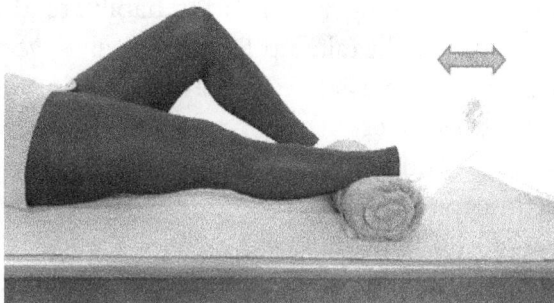

Figure 119: Ankle pump exercises

As discussed earlier, walking and other exercises also help in preventing DVT. Moving your ankle up and down for about four to five minutes and repeating them every hour can go a long way. Also swing your knee 10 to 15 times, gently, while sitting on a high chair (figure 121). These exercises can also be done when you are travelling.

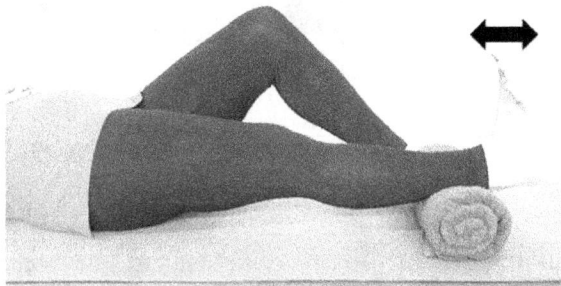

Figure 120: Ankle pump exercise

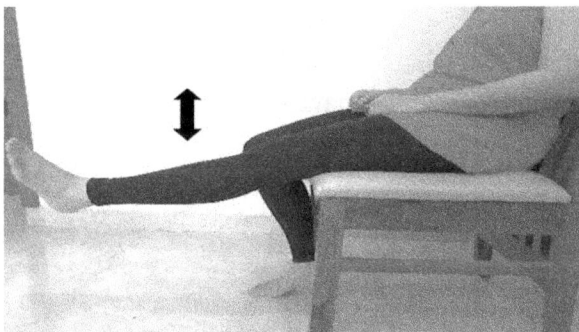

Figure 121: Knee swing

Quadriceps Set Exercises

You can lie down for these exercises. Tighten the thigh muscles and push your thigh and knees down towards the bed (figure 122). Hold it for ten seconds and practice this ten times per set. The complete set must be performed at least four to five times a day.

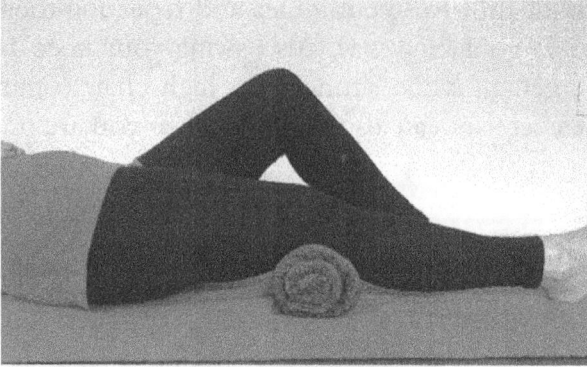

Figure 122: Static quadriceps exercises.

Walking

Walking, one of the essential tasks in our lives, is often not given enough credit. It is the best exercise one can get post hip and knee replacements. Most patients usually start walking within a day or two after surgery.

During the initial four to five days post-surgery, patients are instructed to walk with the help of a walker or two crutches. This may be continued until you are comfortable.

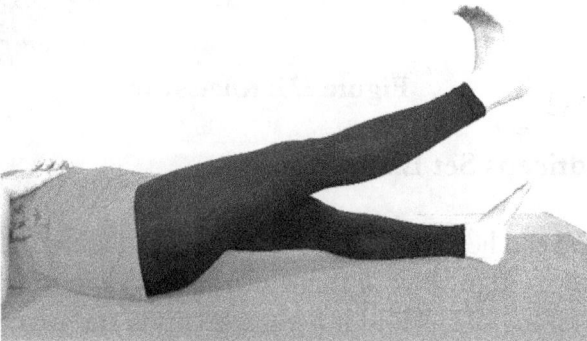

Figure 123: Straight leg rising.

Some patients with both the knee replacements performed together may need it for at least four to five weeks. Again, this depends on the patients' individual capacity. If you are comfortable using a single stick, you can do so after three-four weeks.

Additionally, it is also important not to overwork yourself. Avoid falls and try to match the steps taken by the non-operated leg. Increase the duration and distance of your walking gradually.

Gait Training

It is crucial to learn to walk normally post total knee replacement and total hip replacement. However, this need not be achieved in the very early days post-operation, although, a conscious attempt could make you walk properly much earlier.

You can place the rolls of paper or cloth, as shown (figures 124 and 125). Try to walk by lifting your knee similar to military march past. It would help if you practised this by walking forward as well as sideways.

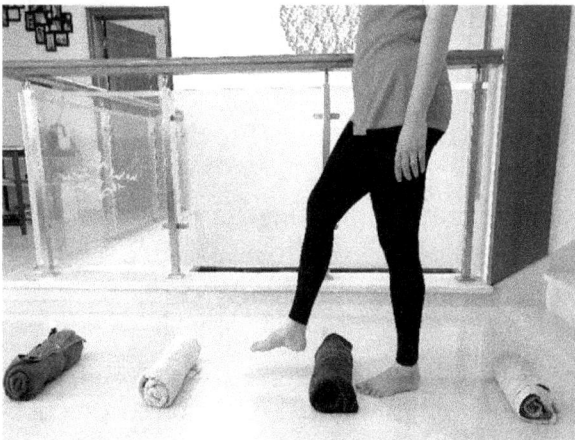

Figure 124: Forward Gait-training

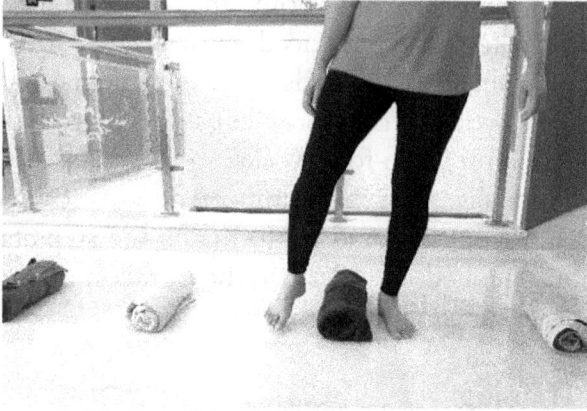

Figure 125: Sideway gait training

Exercise Specific to Total Knee Replacements

There are different types of exercise regimens. Most of them are simple and do not require either machines or a physiotherapist. The purpose of these exercises is to

1) Prevent deep vein thrombosis, as described above
2) Achieve knee bending (flexion)
3) Achieve knee straightening (extension)
4) Gain strength (quadriceps)
5) Improve your walking style

To Achieve Knee Bending (Flexion)

You can practice this lying on your bed. Slowly start bending your knee as much as possible, and when it is bent to its maximum capacity, hold for 10 seconds, and then straighten it again (figure 126).

Make this around ten times per set and practice the entire set four times a day. You can also practice this by sitting on a chair.

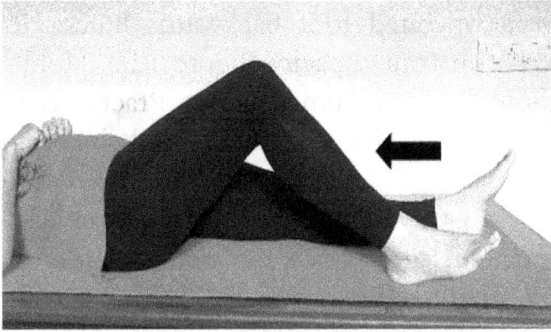

Figure 126: Heal – slide

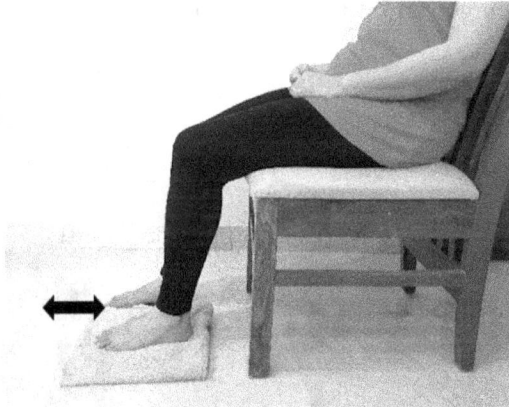

Figure 127: Heel slide with a towel

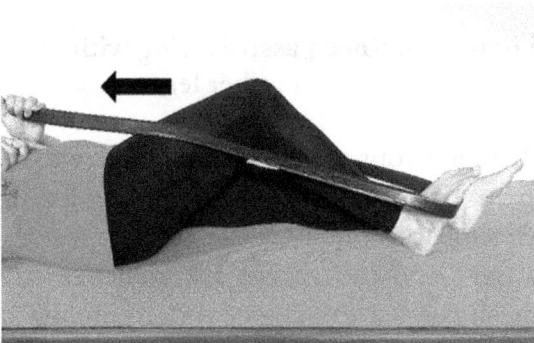

Figure 128: Passive knee bending

Place your foot on a folded towel or a mat and slowly slide your operated foot backwards [under the chair], depending on your capacity (figure 127). Hold it for ten seconds, and do it ten times per set. Practice the entire set four times a day. You can also use a belt to pull the leg (figure 128).

While you are sitting on a chair, you can also use your non operated leg to push the operated leg to improve bending (figure 129).

Additionally, you can practice this by lying down on your stomach. This can be started after two to three weeks post- surgery, when the pain is little better.

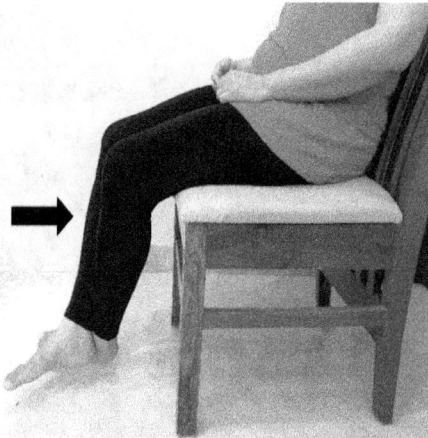

Figure 129: Knee passive swing with the help of another leg

Try bending your operated knee and try to touch your heel to your buttocks (figure 130). Hold it for 10 seconds, and then similar to previous exercises, repeat the set four times a day. You can always ask someone to help you gently push the leg to achieve more bending than what you can do yourself, or you can also use a belt to bend the knee (figure 131).

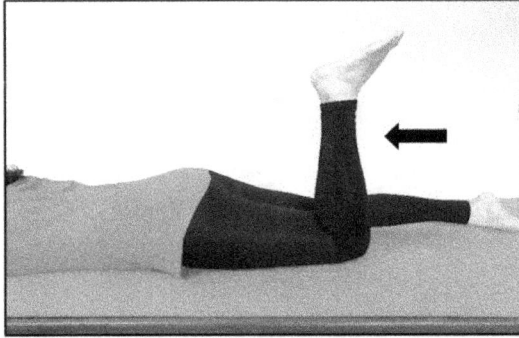

Figure 130: Prone knee bending

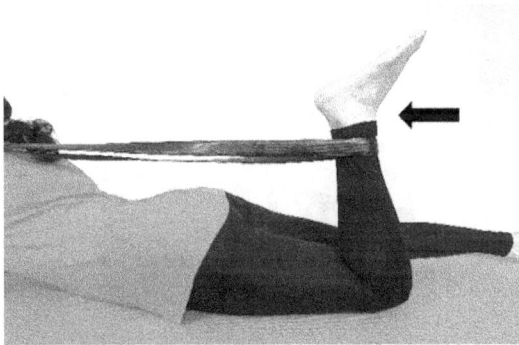

Figure 131: Prone passive knee bending

To Achieve Knee Straightening

Most patients tend to keep their knees slightly bent post-surgery because of the intense pain; however, straightening the knee is particularly important. Please refrain from keeping a pillow under your knee while sleeping. Instead, you can keep a pillow under your foot and press it hard (figure 132). Do all these exercises (of counting till 10) 10 times, and four times a day.

It would help if you also held your leg up while sitting on a chair (figure 133). Use another chair and sit with two kilograms of weight suspended from the knee, as shown in (figure 134).

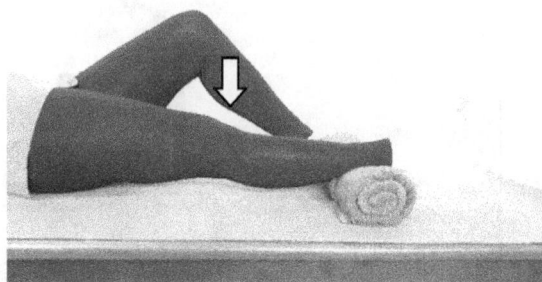

Figure 132: Push the knee down towards bed

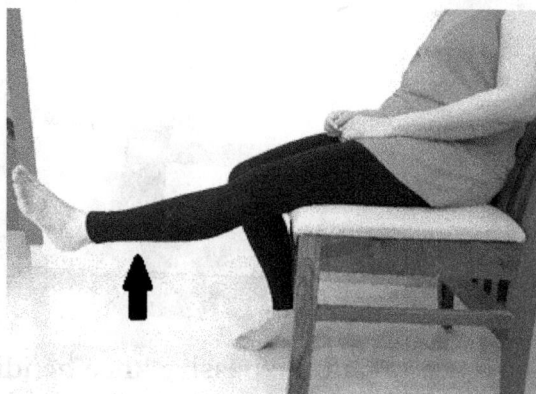

Figure 133: Lift up the knee

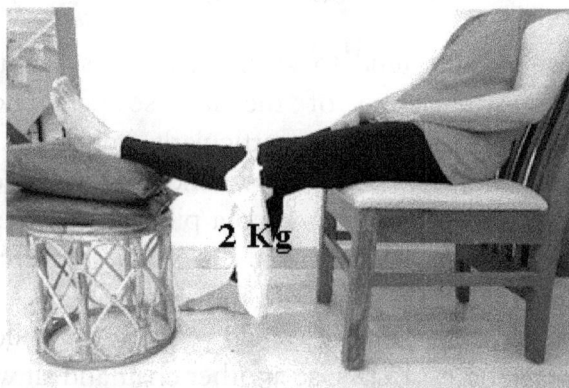

Figure 134: 2 kilograms of weight to straighten the knee

To Gain Strength

The muscles around the knee joint become weak post-surgery, and it is a necessity to exercise to gain back the strength. This weakness is mainly due to reduced activity and intense pain.

However, regaining strength may take a long time. All three exercises described below are done lying down on your back comfortably on a bed. Just like previous exercises, they are a set of ten which has to be repeated four times a day.

• Tighten the thigh muscles as if you are trying to straighten the knee (figure 122).
• Place a small rolled towel under your knee and press (figure 122)
• Raise your leg straight up, to 30 degrees (figure 123). Once you are comfortable, you can add incremental ankle weights, make it a little challenging, and level-up the strength-training. You can add one kilogram to start with and gradually increase to four kgs.

Exercises Specific to Total Hip Replacements

You can start with hip exercises the very next day of the surgery. Very similar to the exercises practised post knee replacements, follow the activities as they are described in the section 'General Exercises.'

When compared to knee replacement, the recovery rate is much faster in hip replacements. You can do all the hip exercises lying on your bed; however, make sure that the cot is neither too low nor too high. Avoid sitting on low sofa beds and chairs.

Buttock Squeeze:

Squeeze both your buttock muscles and hold them tightly for ten seconds. Repeat these steps ten times and practice the set four times a day.

Hip and Knee Bending:

Slide your heel gently towards the buttocks (figure 126). Keep the knee up, pointing straight towards the roof and hold the position for ten seconds, then straighten your knee, and relax for five seconds. Repeat the set of ten four times a day.

Leg Slides:

Leg slides help improve the sideway movements of the hips. For this exercise, lie down comfortably on the bed and keep your knee straight. Now, move your operated leg gently towards the edge of the bed and then bring it back to its original position. Repeat the set of ten, four times a day.

Straight Leg Rises:

These exercises are similar to what has been described in the total knee replacement section (figure 123).

References

1. Neil Artz, Karen T Elvers , Catherine Minns Lowe: Effectiveness of physiotherapy exercise following total knee replacement: systematic review and meta-analysis. BMC Musculoskelet Disord. 2015 Feb 7;16:15.

2. Enhanced Recovery After Surgery (ERAS)-Total hip replacement: New Zealand Orthopaedic Association. (2013). Joint Registry Fourteen Year Report, 1–148.
3. A patient's guide to Total knee replacement. www.rnoh.nhs.uk.
4. Rutherford RW, Jennings JM, Dennis DA. Enhancing Recovery: After total knee arthroplasty: Orthop Clin North Am. 2017 Oct;48(4):391-400.
5. Chen H, Li S, Ruan T, Liu L, Fang L: Is it necessary to perform prehabilitation exercise for patients undergoing total knee arthroplasty: meta-analysis of randomized controlled trials. Phys Sportsmed. 2018 Feb;46(1):36-43.

DR. NARAYAN HULSE

14
LIFE AFTER JOINT REPLACEMENTS

Patients who undergo joint replacement surgeries can lead a healthy life and take part in most of the recreational activities. Even though pain relief is the primary goal of these operations, many patients improve their activity level and also their quality of life. However, time taken to achieve these goals varies depending on a variety of physical and emotional factors like age, general health, attitude, social support, mental abilities, etc.

Climbing Stairs

Basic stair climbing is possible within a week after knee or hip replacement. However, it might take a longer time than expected if you are weak and are suffering from other medical conditions.

Make a note of these points. While walking up the stairs, use your operated leg first (figure 135). Take one step at a time initially, and increase the speed gradually. While coming down the stairs use the non-operated leg first. Then follow the sequence, as shown in figure 136.

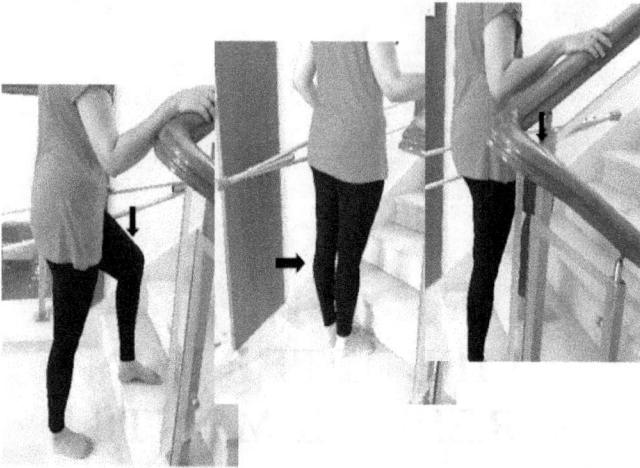

Figure 135: Sequence of climbing stairs: right is the operated knee

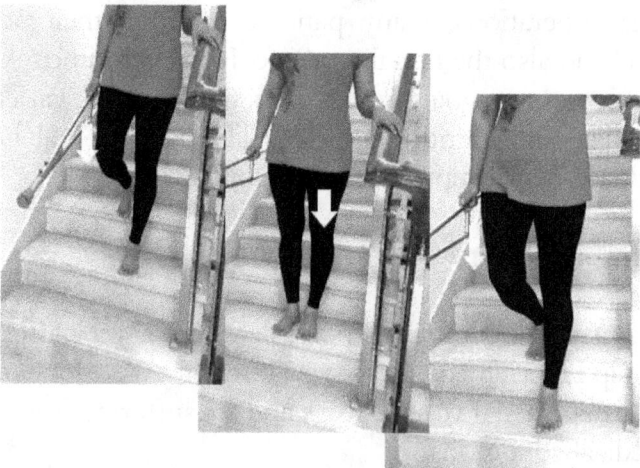

Figure 136: Sequence of walking down the stairs: right is the operated knee

Sitting and Standing

As mentioned earlier, make sure to use higher chairs and toilet seats; they should be at least of your knee height. You could use cushions on normal chairs and toilet seat elevators on the commodes to increase the height. This arrangement may be needed for six to eight weeks after surgery.

While sitting down, first touch the chair with the back of your thigh and then leave the walking aids. Slowly hold the armrests of the chair using both your hands. Stretch your operated leg forward and then lower yourself down on the chair.

Similarly, while standing up, place your hands on the armrest first. Place your body weight on the non-operated leg and keep your operated leg stretched forward. Rise slowly and maintain the balance on your feet. Now reach out to your walking aids.

Note: Never lean on the walking aids to pull yourself up.

Bath and Shower

You must be careful about the accidental falls while taking a shower. Once the stitches are removed, say in about 14 days, you can soak the knee in soap and water without any protective cover on the wound. When you are in the hospital, nurses will help you to clean your body, usually with a sponge bath.

When you are mobile with a walker, usually in about four to five days after surgery, you can shower directly over the waterproof dressing. However, it is better to seek help for at least three to four weeks. Using a bathtub might have to wait for about six to eight weeks.

Wearing Clothes

You can start wearing normal clothes once you are discharged; opt for comfortable clothing. While wearing trousers or similar outfits, put in on the operated leg first. You can also use reachers, dressing sticks, sock aid, and long shoehorn if needed, although most patients manage without these aids.

Getting In and Out of Cars

Park the car in a safe place, with enough room for you to reach the vehicle along with your walking aid. It would help if you initially sat on the front passenger seat. Push the car seat as rear as possible so that you will have enough space to stretch your legs. While sitting down, place your hand on the seat, lower yourself, and then sit comfortably facing the car door. Then turn forward while gently bringing your legs inside the car. Position yourself until you are sitting comfortably (figures 137, 138 and 139). Reverse these steps while getting out of the vehicle.

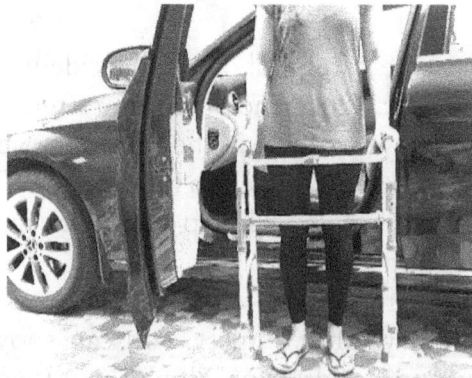

Figure 137: Step 1: Approach the front passenger's seat as shown

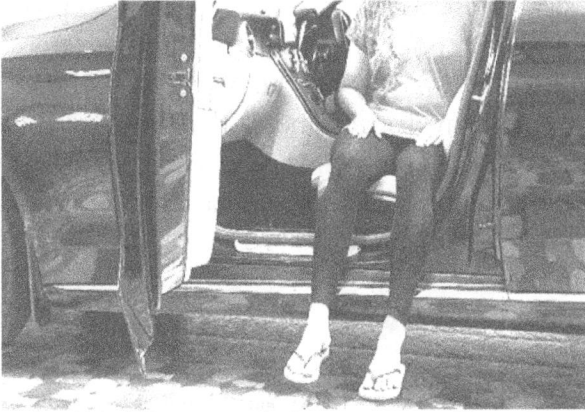

Figure 138: Then gently lower yourself on the seat

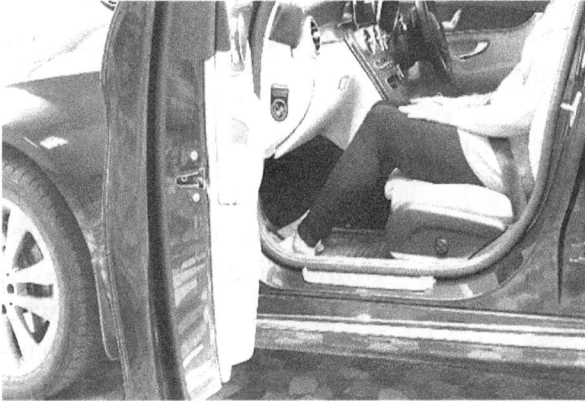

Figure 139: Then turn gently to face front

Travelling

Avoid long-distance and non-essential travel as much as possible, until four to six weeks post-surgery. Besides being uncomfortable, sitting for a long time also increases the chances of deep vein thrombosis, especially the long-haul air travels. However, if you have to travel due to unavoidable circumstances, don't forget to take the necessary precautions, like taking prophylactic medications, continuing ankle pump exercises, and intermittent walking inside the plane. Also, the implant in your joints may trigger metal detectors at the airport security check. You may want to carry a card or a letter describing the presence of a metal implant in your body issued by your hospital.

Driving

You will be able to drive usually in six to eight weeks after surgery. However, consider driving only when if you have good movements and are pain-free. You may want to confirm with your insurance and driving authorities about the legal requirements for driving in your state/country.

Job and Work

Patients who undergo joint replacements are mostly elderly and retired from active occupations. They can resume all household chores after six to eight weeks.

You can also return to work in about eight to ten weeks if it is desk/in-office jobs. It would be best to avoid manual jobs requiring frequent squatting and kneeling.

Sports and Other Activities

Returning to most of the sports activities is possible after three months. However, this is possible only if you have practised these sports before your surgery. Taking to a new sport might get tricky.

Walking, swimming, cycling, and golfing are easily achievable. You can also participate in other sports, but make sure you are not causing undue strain on the replaced joint and do not twist the hip joint. Avoid all impact and contact sports like football, basketball, rugby, etc. The various forms of dancing, especially with slow moves suitable for the elderly age group, can be easily performed.

Regular sexual activity is possible after you have recovered completely. Remember, you should be a passive partner while you are recovering. Once recovered, there is no need to take precautions for knee replacements. However, any painful positioning and extreme joint movements should be avoided to prevent dislocations of the hip joints.

References

1) F. Canovas, L. Dagneaux: Quality of life after total knee arthroplasty Orthopaedics & Traumatology: Surgery & Research 104 (2018) S41–S46.
2) Before, During & After Hip and Knee Replacement Surgery: http://vch.eduhealth.ca.

15
HOW LONG DOES A JOINT REPLACEMENT LAST?

Survival of an implant is the duration from the date of primary surgery to its failure resulting in revision surgery. In general, 80 to 90 per cent of the joint replacements last for about 20 years.

To support this speculation, we have strong data from millions of people who have undergone surgery all over the world in the last seventy years.

These survival data are obtained from several national joint registries. The Swedish Knee Arthroplasty was established as the first national arthroplasty registry in 1975, followed by the Swedish Hip Arthroplasty Registry in 1979. These registries help in identifying implants that are performing poorly at an early stage and also help to take remedial actions.

Survival of a joint replacement depends on a variety of factors. Data from joint registries have shown that more than 80% of the knee prostheses survive until the 25 years follow-up. On the other hand, the risk of failure leading to revision knee replacement in ten years after the primary surgery is about 5%.

Common Causes of Failure

- Loosening of the implant- 29.8%
- Infection- 14.8%
- Pain - 9.5%.

After hip replacements, similar outcomes are reported.

Bayliss and colleagues had reported 20-year survival of 85% of the implants from the analysis of 63,158 patients with a maximum follow-up of 20 years.

After 15 years, 89.4% of hip replacements had survived out of 215,676 hips studied from both the Australian and Finnish registries.

After 20 years, 70.2% were intact (95% CI 69.7 to 70.7; 73,057 hips from the Finnish registry). After 25 years, 57.9% were still intact (95% CI 57.1 to 58.7; 51,359 hips from the Finnish registry).

Using available arthroplasty registry data, we estimate that about three-quarters of hip replacements last 15–20 years and just over half of hip replacements last for 25 years in patients with osteoarthritis.

Several factors influence the longevity of a joint replacement. While some of the elements are related to your body and general health, others are related to the technique and types of joint replacements.

- Rate of revision decreases with age. Younger patients have early revisions.
- Men have higher rates of revision than women. Cumulative Risk of Revision (CRR) in men aged > 75 years is 2%, ten years post-operatively, whereas in those aged < 55 years it is 12%.

- Obese patients have higher complications and failed joint replacements.
- Patients with rheumatoid arthritis who undergo TKA have higher rate of infection leading to revision, especially in men.
- Partial arthroplasty, including unicompartmental, patellofemoral, bicompartmental, uni-spacer, and partial resurfacing, have a higher rate of revisions than TKA.
- Risk of revision is substantially increased with the use of uncemented compared with cemented implants in knee replacements.
- Computer navigated TKAs performed in patients aged < 65 years are less likely to require revision for loosening or osteolysis, according to some studies.
- Finally, the outcome is better if the operation is undertaken by a surgeon who performs a large number of joint replacements. This has been reported several times.
- Prostheses using high cross-linked polyethylene (XLPE) have a lower rate of revision compared with those using non-cross-linked polyethylene.

Reference:

1) Jonathan T Evans, Robert W Walker, Jonathan P Evans, et al: How long does a knee replacement last? A systematic review and meta-analysis of case series and national registry reports with more than 15 years of follow-up. 2019 Feb 16;393(10172):655-663.

2) Sharkey PF, Hozack WJ, Rothman RH, Shastri S, Jacoby SM. Insall Award paper. Why are total knee arthroplasties failing today? Clin Orthop Relat Res 2002;404:7– 13.

3) Vertullo CJ, Lewis PL, Graves S, Kelly L, Lorimer M, Myers P: Twelve-Year Outcomes of an Oxinium Total Knee Replacement Compared with the Same Cobalt-

Chromium Design: An Analysis of 17,577 Prostheses from the Australian Orthopaedic Association. National Joint Replacement Registry. J Bone Joint Surg Am. 2017 Feb 15;99(4):275-283.

4) Postler A, Lützner C, Beyer F, Tille E, Lützner J:Analysis of Total Knee Arthroplasty revision causes. BMC Musculoskelet Disord. 2018 Feb 14;19(1):55.

16
DEALING WITH A FAILED JOINT REPLACEMENT

A failed joint replacement need not be the end of the world. Joint replacement surgery is one of the most successful surgical procedures, and over 90% of patients need no further treatment during their entire lifetime. However, those patients with failed joint replacements may need revision joint replacements.

In the last two decades, the revision joint replacements are being performed in large numbers, and their results are improving tremendously because of the advances in surgical techniques and implant materials.

For a patient, failed replacement is of great concern as this may lead to pain, multiple hospital visits, further surgical operations, and expenditure. However, we must realize that there is an underlying risk with every medical procedure you undergo.

If there is a problem, then it should be resolved with the best available methods and technology. Your joint should be assessed thoroughly before any further treatment is advocated.

- When you notice unusual pain, swelling or deterioration in the function of the joint, you should see your surgeon.

- There need not be a mechanical fault all the time to cause pain.

- Many people who undergo a joint replacement may need a long time to reach an optimum outcome. It could be even 12 months before your knee is fully healed. During this time, no major intervention should be performed unless there is objective evidence to suggest a problem.

- Joint replacement is an artificial implant. This may not feel as natural as a native knee or exactly the way you would like it to be. You should know that the purpose of a joint replacement is to relieve you from the pain and help you perform all the normal daily activities without being dependent on painkillers.

- Some of the pain may also be radiating from the other joints and nerves. For example, hip pain after a hip replacement may be a referred pain arising from your spine. Pain in the total knee may be from the hip or spine.

- Knee replacement will relieve the pain originating from the knee. It is natural to feel the pain and ache in the leg occasionally like everyone else. But this pain should not stay for a long time, and it definitely should not be originating from the replaced joint.

- If you have mild pain, simple exercises and medications should be able to manage it; a surgical procedure is not required.

- If there is no demonstrable mechanical problem in the joint replacement, re-surgery may fail again. So, it is not generally preferred.

- A small number of patients may continue to have a variable amount of pain without any demonstrable issues in the joint replacement. This leads to a lot of dilemmas in further management.

- A set of investigations may be needed before we arrive at a diagnosis. Blood tests, X-rays, culture test from the fluid removed from your knee, a CT scan and occasionally a radioisotope bone scan may be needed.
- Depending on the cause of the pain, you may need appropriate interventions, which could be medications, pain clinic consultations, physical therapies, and rarely further surgery.

Several options are available to treat failed joints. These surgeries and other options can be difficult and expensive. Commonly used options are revision or re-surgery, excision or removal of components and leaving with false joints, arthrodesis, or fusion of both the bones and variety of braces and pain-relieving medications.

References:

1) Zachary C Lum, Alvin K Shieh, Lawrence D Dorr: Why total knees fail-A modern perspective review. World J Orthop 2018 April 18; 9(4): 60-64.

2) Khan M, Osman K, Green G, Haddad FS: The epidemiology of failure in total knee arthroplasty: avoiding your next revision. Bone Joint J. 2016 Jan;98-B(1 Suppl A):105-12.

3) Delanois RE, Mistry JB, Gwam CU, Mohamed NS, Choksi US, Mont MA. Current Epidemiology of Revision Total Knee Arthroplasty in the United States. J Arthroplasty. 2017, Sep;32(9):2663-2668.

4) Gwam CU, Mistry JB, Mohamed NS, Thomas M, Bigart KC, Mont MA, Delanois RE. Current Epidemiology of Revision Total Hip Arthroplasty in the United States: National Inpatient Sample 2009 to

2013. J Arthroplasty. 2017 Jul;32(7):2088 2092.

5) Bozic KJ, Kurtz SM, Lau E, Ong K, Vail TP, Berry DJ: The epidemiology of revision total hip arthroplasty in the United States. J Bone Joint Surg Am. 2009 Jan;91(1):128-33.

Case 30: Her Hip Replacement Failed After 22-years, Calling for a Re-Surgery

Mrs. Kamini (name changed), a lady in her late 70s, had undergone a successful hip replacement 22-years-ago. She started experiencing a slight pain in her hip recently and the pain had intensified over the last six months. She had also developed an infection, which resulted in pus pouring out of the hip.

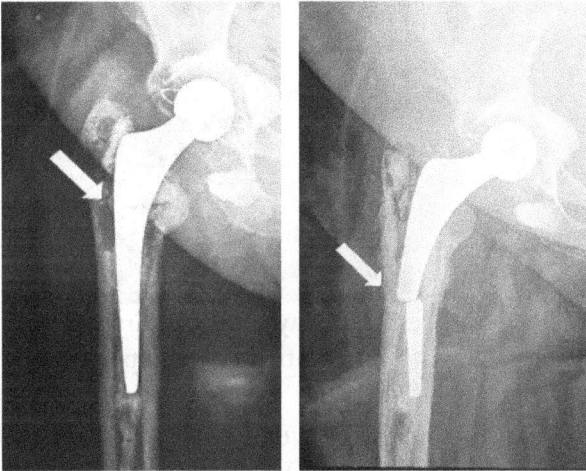

Figure 140: (a)Loose hip replacement, which ultimately broke (b)

She consulted several doctors regarding this condition, and most of them advised her to get a two-stage revision hip replacement done. However, she hesitated to go forward as she was worried about the risks associated with it.

Giving in to her fear, she ended up opting for an unscientific therapy in another hospital. She received a small surgery to evacuate the pus and was put on prolonged antibiotic treatment. For one thing, this method is doomed to fail because an implant that is loose and infected needs to be removed. That is the only way to deal with this problem. So, as expected, within a few days, the pus started pouring out again.

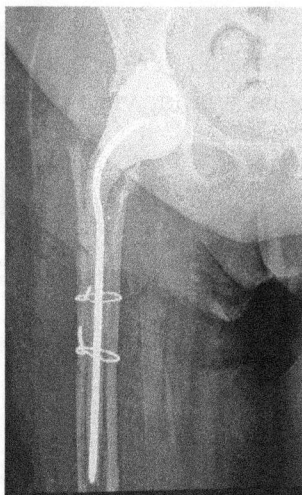

Figure 141: X-ray after the first stage with antibiotic cement spacer

Mrs. Kamini further developed severe pain in her hip and was unable to walk. An X-ray taken at this point showed a broken hip implant and further loosening of the hip replacement. This is when she decided to go for the proposed two-staged surgery.

In the first stage of the operation, we removed all the implants and bone cement. Her hip joint was surgically cleaned, and then a cement spacer with a large dose of antibiotics was placed.

Mrs. Kamini was then sent home, and the antibiotic treatment was continued at home. Luckily, Mrs Kamini stayed with her family, her greatest social support. So, she did not have to worry about anything and could take care of herself.

She returned to the hospital in eight weeks for the removal of spacer and insertion of a new hip replacement. This way, she recovered well and got rid of her pain, pus, and immobility.

17
COST OF THE JOINT REPLACEMENTS

The cost of joint replacement surgery varies significantly from hospital to hospital and place to place. Your total bill includes:

a) Hospital expenses for conducting the surgery such as wards, operation theatre, nursing services, and food.

b) Cost of the implant used. They are priced extremely high because they are usually imported.

c) Fees paid to the surgeons, anaesthetists, and their team.

d) Consultation fees of other doctors like cardiologists and physicians.

e) Investigations such as blood tests, ECG, and x rays.

f) Your total expenses may also depend on the number of days you stay at the hospital and also the type of ward you stay in. Usually, deluxe or en-suite rooms are costlier in comparison to sharing rooms and general wards.

g) Unanticipated equipment used in the treatment or other inevitable situations where a patient is in dire need of intensive care unit might also escalate the charges.

Although most hospitals provide you with an estimate of charges, it may not be very accurate. Even if you are covered with insurance, you must understand the whole process and be aware of these out-of-the-pocket expenses.

So, Is It Cheaper to Live Without a Joint Replacement?

This is a very tricky question to answer. Indeed, joint replacements may not be affordable to those who are uninsured; however, if one chooses not to get the replacement done, living with reduced mobility can also lead to significant financial losses.

A knee replacement helps you by relieving the pain and saves you from costly pain medications that have to be taken every day. Additionally, if a person is independent and can take care of himself, it will reduce the burden on the family and the society in general. This is very true in cases where the patient is the sole breadwinner of the family.

On the whole, if you calculate several other social and medical factors, your entire life will be more expensive if you are living with an arthritic knee pain instead of considering than a knee replacement.

What Is the Cost of The Implants?

The price of the implants varies from company to company. To prevent unreasonable profiteering, some of the states have fixed a ceiling price for these implants. For example, in India, the costs of the implants are as below. This data is as of 2019.

Ceiling Prices on Primary Knee Implants in India-2019
(Prices in INR)

Component	Material	Ceiling Price without tax	Ceiling Price with tax (5%)
Femoral Component	Titanium Alloy	₹38,740	₹40,677
Femoral Component	Oxidized Zirconium	₹38,740	₹40,677
Femoral Component	Hi-Flex	₹25,860	₹27,153
Femoral Component	Cobalt Chromium	₹24,090	₹25,295
Tibial Component	Titanium Alloy	₹24,280	₹25,494
Tibial Component	Oxidized Zirconium	₹24,280	₹25,494
Tibial Component	Cobalt Chromium	₹16,990	₹17,840
Articulating Surface	Any Material	₹9,550	₹10,028
Patella	Any Material	₹4,090	₹4,295
Tibial Tray + Insert	Polyethylene or crosslinked polyethylene or high crosslinked polyethylene	₹12,960	₹13,608

Tibial Tray + Insert	Tibial: Metallic Insert: Polyethylene or crosslinked polyethylene or high crosslinked polyethylene or any other material	₹26,546	₹27,873

Ceiling Prices on Revision Knee Implants in India-2019
(Prices in INR)

Component	Material	Ceiling price with tax	Ceiling price with tax (5%)
Femoral Component	Any Material	₹62,770	₹65,909
Tibial Component	Any Material	₹31,220	₹32,781
Articulating Surface	Any Material	₹15,870	₹16,664
Patella	Any Material	₹4,090	₹4,295

Approximate total charges in different countries for joint replacements is listed below (indicative only: can vary from hospital to hospital)

Country	Total knee	Total hip
India	₹2 to ₹4 Lakh, (INR)	₹2 to ₹4 Lakh (INR)
USA (USD)	$30 to 49,500	$35 to 50,000
UK (GBP)	£11400 to 15400	£8,500 to 16,800
Australia (AUD)	$17,797 to 30,285	$19,439 to 42,007
Singapore (USD)	$16,000	$14000 to 16000
Italy (USD)	$22,729	$21000
Canada (CAD)	$10,000 to $35,000	$10,000 to 35,000
Malaysia (USD)	$7000	$8,000

References:

1) Weinstein AM, Rome BN, Reichmann WM, et al. Estimating the burden of total knee replacement in the United States. J Bone Joint Surg Am 2013; 95:385–392 3.

2) Palsis JA, Brehmer TS, Pellegrini VD, Drew JM, Sachs BL: The Cost of Joint Replacement: Comparing Two Approaches to Evaluating Costs of Total Hip and Knee Arthroplasty.J Bone Joint Surg Am. 2018 Feb 21;100(4):326-333.

3) Kamaruzaman H, Kinghorn P, Oppong R. Cost-effectiveness of surgical interventions for the management of osteoarthritis: a systematic review of the literature. BMC Musculoskelet Disord. 2017 May 10;18(1):183.

4) Molloy IB, Martin BI, Moschetti WE, Jevsevar DS. Effects of the Length of Stay on the cost of total knee and Total Hip Arthroplasty from 2002 to 2013. J Bone Joint Surg Am. 2017 Mar 1;99(5):402- 407.

Case 31: She Travelled All the Way from Nigeria for Both Knee Replacements to Relieve Knock-Knee

Sixty-six-year-old Mary (name changed) from Nigeria, suffering from severe pain in both knees, had developed progressive inward bending of both the knees called 'knock-knees.' She weighed around 115 kgs, although she had left no stones unturned trying to reduce her weight. Given this severe bending and obesity, she was indeed a high-risk candidate for surgery.

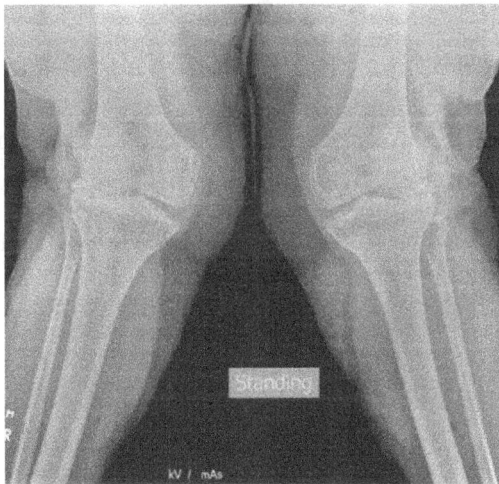

Figure 142: Knock knees

However, she met with one of our patients who had undergone both knee replacements a couple of years ago, and on recommendation, she flew all the way to India for her replacement surgery. After all general medical assessment, she underwent staged knee replacements.

She recovered surprisingly well and also consulted a bariatric surgeon regarding her obesity. However, to her surprise, she could walk well and even exercise to reduce weight.

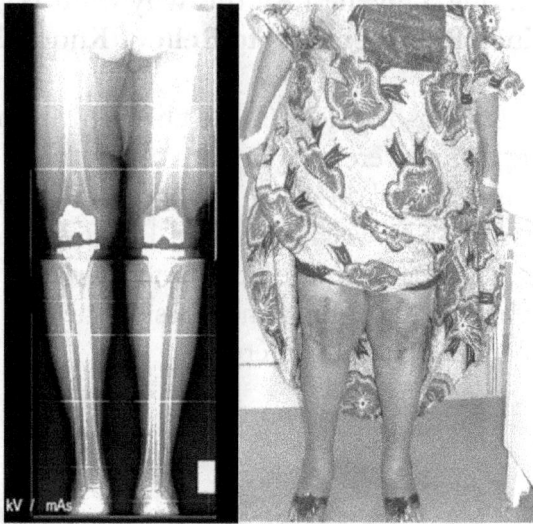

Figure 143: Long radiograph and straight knees after surgery

Within 12 months, she lost about 15 kgs and is looking to reduce more at the moment.

18
MODERN TECHNOLOGIES AND FUTURE DEVELOPMENTS

Summary:
Several innovations such as computer navigation, custom knees, kinematic concepts, 3D printing, and robotic joint replacements are available and have shown variable success and acceptance. However, there is no need to rush behind a new technology just because it is well publicised, commercially.

Medical innovations are true life-changers, especially the inventions made in the joint replacements sector. However, many of these innovative products might not have gone through vigorous medical trials and may lack long term, real-time experience on an adequate number of patients. This, in turn, makes it difficult for the patients and even the surgeons to choose a product without bias.

However, there are some institutions like Food and Drug Administration [FDA] in the USA, the National

Institute for Clinical Excellence [NICE] guidelines in the UK, and similar other regulatory bodies worldwide that can help you choose by scientifically analyzing the products.

Implants used inside your body should be safe, cost-effective, and successful in a large number of patients over many years. Hence, you should never blindly trust these technologies just because they are 'latest.' Although promoted well, these products might not suit you.

Computer-Aided Navigation

Performing knee and hip joint replacement involves placing the prosthetic components accurately with respect to your leg's alignment. Accurate placement of the components is vital for achieving adequate function and life of the artificial joint.

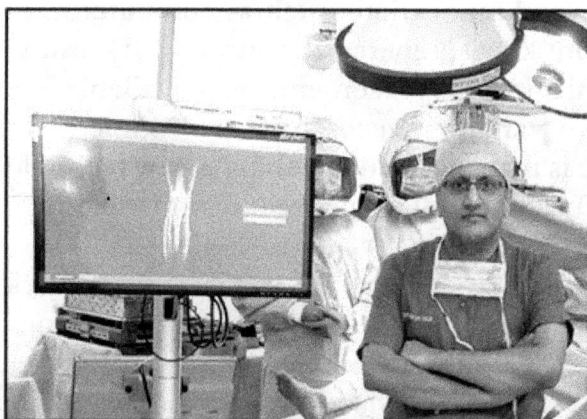

Figure 144: Author with the computer navigation system

Conventionally, this is achieved using mechanical instruments called jigs, which are used to measure various angles and axis. However, it is important to note that mechanical measurement using jigs and the bare eye can recognize only up to a certain limit.

Computer navigation was introduced in 1994 with a plan to achieve higher accuracy of component placement and proper limb alignment.

In this method, the computer receives dynamic signals from the knee using trackers. This helps the surgeon cut the bone and fix the components accurately and correct the limb alignment.

Several studies have now shown that computer navigation is excellent in achieving the precise placement of the knee components. Navigation is extremely useful in correcting some of the problematic knee replacements such as previous fractures (extra-articular deformities) and in the presence of previous metal implants around the knee. But navigation adds to the cost and surgical time of the surgery.

A large study from the Australian joint registry showed decreased failures and revisions of knee replacements performed using computer navigations.

However, most of the other large studies and joint registries found no benefit of using the navigation in terms of function, pain, complications, and survival of the implant and revisions.

Custom Knees

Also called patient-specific instrumentations or patient-specific cutting blocks, this method involves an MRI or a CT scan of your knee taken several weeks before the surgery. These scans are sent to the manufacturing company where cutting jigs are prepared using the 3D images.

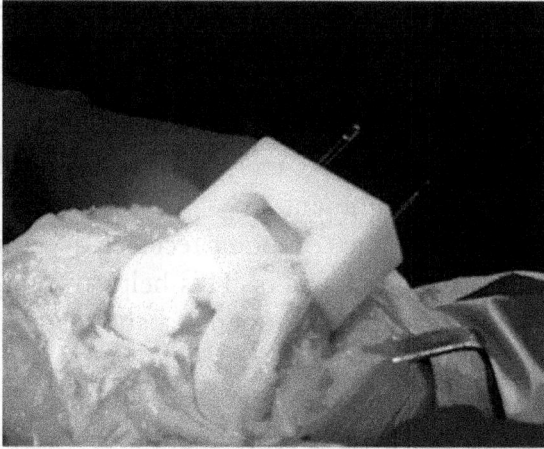

Figure 145: Custom instrumentation during surgery

During the surgery, these jigs are placed on the surface of your knee bones and are then cut using the slots in the jigs. These jigs can also reduce the number of mechanical instruments needed in the operation theatre, thereby reducing the operation theatre inventory and their processing.

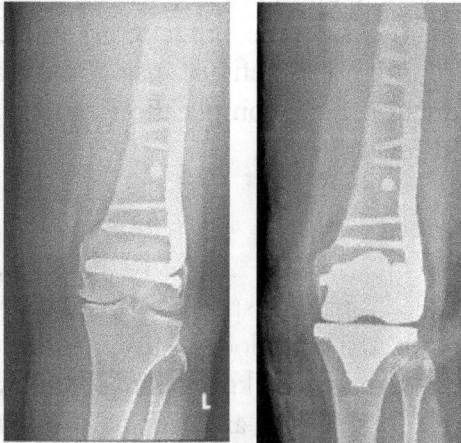

Figure 146: TKR without removing old metals (used to treat a fracture earlier) using custom instrumentation

However, this technique is slowly losing its popularity in recent times, given the additional time required to manufacture these jigs before surgery. The added costs, and lesser accuracy of component placement compared to computer navigation are a few other reasons.

Kinematic Knee Alignment

While performing a total knee replacement, your surgeon will place the prosthesis in correct alignment with respect to the axis of your leg from hip to ankle. In a standard knee replacement, this is a straight line called the mechanical axis. In this technique of mechanical alignment, your knee is replaced in such a way that your leg is completely straight, and the joint line will be exactly perpendicular to the axis of the leg.

Despite achieving good alignment using the mechanical alignment techniques, a significant number of the patients (15– 20%) may not be completely satisfied with their artificial knee. In the kinematic concepts, the knee is not completely brought back to a straight line but restored to the pre-arthritic alignment of that particular patient. Although some surgeons had started using this method way back in 2006, it has not been administered in large numbers. Thus, more scientific studies with a large number of people and long-term follow-ups are required to evaluate further the advantages and disadvantages of the kinematic alignment in total knee replacement.

3D Printing Technology:

Joint replacements need planning and preoperative preparations. This is critical, especially in complicated cases with major bone loss. Sometimes, a variety of reconstruction methods and special implants may have to be used to compensate for the loss of bone stock during revision hip replacements. This planning is impossible with simple X-rays. Hence a 3D model of your hip is created using a CT scan, which is used for the planning and selection of implants and other reconstructive options.

Note: This technique is not necessary in simple cases. Also, it is expensive and time-consuming.

Robotic Joint Replacements:

There have been tremendous improvements seen in the robotic world over the years, so much so that even in the medical field, robots have been developed to perform complex surgical tasks. There have been many robotic-assisted joint replacement techniques available for knee, hip, and partial knee replacements, at the moment.

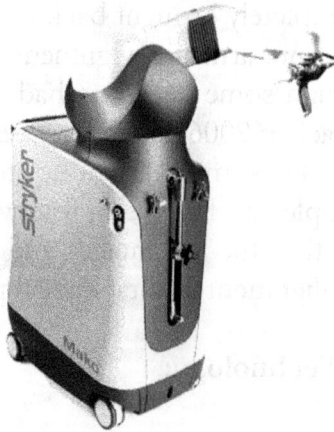

Figure 147: MAKO total knee robotic arm (Stryker, Kalamazoo, MI)

However, this should not cause any concern as the surgeon primarily performs the surgery, and all that the robot does is to assist the operator in performing critical procedures accurately. The robotic arm helps the surgeon perform the surgery more precisely.

Here's what happens in robot-assisted surgery:

1. The patient will undergo a CT scan before the surgery.
2. The surgeon will then analyse the 3D images with the help of special program associated with the robotic machine. This helps to ensure the correct sizing and positioning of the components of your artificial knee.
3. During surgery, robotic arms control the depth and extent of bone cuts. They also prevent any accidental damage to the vital structures, ligaments, and other soft tissues. This technique will enable accurate component positioning along with the prevention of inadvertent damage to the surrounding structures.

Several studies conducted in the past have shown early evidence to prove that robotic partial knee replacements are indeed superior in terms of component positioning, function and failed procedures needing revisions.

However, at the moment, there is no conclusive evidence that proves that robotic knee and hip replacements are better than conventional techniques.

Robotic machines are prohibitively expensive, and more research is needed to evaluate if the robotic joint replacement is effective to improve the outcomes.

Reference:

1) Jorgensen NB, McAuliffe M, Orschulok T, Lorimer MF, de Steiger R: Major Aseptic Revision Following Total Knee Replacement: A Study of 478,081 Total Knee Replacements from the Australian Orthopaedic Association National Joint Replacement Registry. J Bone Joint Surg Am. 2019 Feb 20;101(4):302-310.

2) Kayani B, Konan S, Ayuob A, Onochie E, Al-Jabri T, Haddad FS: Robotic technology in total knee arthroplasty: a systematic review. EFORT Open Rev. 2019 Oct 1;4(10):611- 61.

3) Koh IJ, Park IJ, Lin CC, Patel NA, Chalmers CE, Maniglio M, McGarry MH, Lee TQ: Kinematically aligned total knee arthroplasty reproduces native patellofemoral biomechanics during deep knee flexion, Knee Surg Sports Traumatol Arthroscopy. 2019 May;27(5):1520-1528.

4) Zagra L. Advances in hip arthroplasty surgery: what is justified? EFORT Open Rev. 2017 May 11;2(5):171-178.

5) J Jones CW, Jerabek SA: Current Role of Computer Navigation in Total Knee Arthroplasty. J Arthroplasty. 2018 Jul;33(7):1989-1993.

FREQUENTLY ASKED QUESTIONS

Before surgery

1. How common is joint replacement surgery?

Currently, joint replacement is one of the most commonly performed orthopaedic surgeries, with millions of people receiving new joints every year. In the USA, about 1.4 million joint replacements are carried out every year, and as of 2017, the number of primary hip and knee replacement surgeries in the UK had reached 91,698 and 102,177, respectively.

In India, more than 2,00,000 joints are replaced every year. As this surgery is not a new procedure, the medical experience is large enough to advocate the procedure in those patients who are suffering from severe joint pain.

2. What is the upper age limit for joint replacement surgery?

There is no upper age limit for joint replacement surgery. Rather than the patient's chronological age, his physiological age (reflecting general health) is more important. Patients should be fit enough to sustain the operation and anaesthesia; a team of doctors will assess this.

3. What is the lower age limit for a joint replacement surgery?

A successful joint replacement can last only for 20 years on average. If the surgery is performed on an older person, it may last his entire life.

However, if conducted on a younger person, it may fail during his lifetime, needing revision surgeries and sometimes multiple revisions.

Revision surgeries are complicated and have less favourable outcomes. Hence, joint replacement surgery is generally avoided in younger patients.

However, in recent times, with increasing technology and research, more and more younger patients are receiving joint replacements. This is advocated only for patients who are suffering from severe pain and limitations in daily living activities.

4. What are the situations when I should not have a joint replacement despite having severe pain?

These situations are called medical contraindications. You should not have a joint replacement surgery if you are suffering from an infection of that joint or anywhere else in the body. The surgery should also be avoided if —

- The muscles of that particular joint are weak
- If the blood supply is poor
- If you are suffering from a severe illness, as your body might not agree with the administered anaesthesia.

5. Which medicine is to be stopped before surgery?

Usually, all the blood thinners are stopped five to seven days before the surgery. If you are taking women-hormones, they should be stopped much early after a consultation with a physician. Some surgeons also advise stopping rheumatoid medications.

6. When does a patient get admitted to the hospital?

Most of the centers admit their patient a day before the surgery for routine evaluations. However, if the patient has completed his/her pre-operative assessment, they can be admitted on the same day as the surgery

7. What are the tests conducted before surgery?

A set of blood tests are conducted before the surgery to assess the patient's general health — ECG, Chest X-ray and an ECHO cardiogram are commonly undertaken. The patient may require other tests and consultations with different specialists depending on his/her health status.

8. Is a joint replacement surgery safe if the patient has diabetes?

Type 2 diabetes is prevalent in countries like India. The strict control of blood sugar level is essential before surgery, to prevent complications.

However, patients with diabetes undergo joint replacement surgery very commonly without any complications.

9. Is a joint replacement surgery safe after heart surgery?

Patients undergoing joint replacement surgery may have some cardiac illness, and as most of the patients are quite old, this is very much expected.

Some patients might have undergone heart-related medical procedures. Most of these patients can receive joint replacement surgery if their cardiac condition is stable. These patients will undergo a thorough evaluation by a cardiologist before the surgery.

10. Is a joint replacement surgery safe in patients suffering from blood pressure?

Joints replacements are performed routinely in patients suffering from hypertension. So, the blood pressure has to be strictly controlled prior to surgery; a general physician usually assesses the patients before surgery.

11. Are there a different variety of joints depending on your functional need?

No. There has been a considerable demand lately to develop more functional and long-lasting knee replacements. High flexion design, rotating flatform, and gender-specific design come with great promise and commercial promotions.

However, most of them have neither changed the results nor the complications over a period of time.

12. Can I sit on the floor after surgery?

After a knee replacement, some patients may be able to sit on the floor cross-legged. However, this should be avoided as much as possible because the force generated on your knees might end up damaging your artificial knees.

13. Will I require an MRI or a CT scan?

No, they aren't usually required unless a patient has

unusual anatomy due to previous trauma or other diseases. Scans are required for some of the new techniques like image-guided navigation, customized instrumentation, and robotic knee replacements.

14. What is a custom-made knee?

These are customized instrumentation and patient-specific instrumentations. Specific instruments are manufactured using your scans performed a few weeks before surgery. While this was designed to increase the accuracy of component placement, results have revealed that custom-made knee is not that superior to conventional methods. They are not that popular in recent times.

15. Is there a special knee implant required if I want to squat on the floor or do yoga?

Contrary to the popular belief and commercial advertisements, there are no such implants in the world specific to the above function.

During Surgery

16. How is the implant affixed in the body?

Metal implants are manufactured in small incremental sizes to suit everybody. Implants of all the sizes will be available in the operation theatre every time a joint replacement is performed. These metal implants are commonly fixed to the bone using bone cement (PMMA). This is called 'cemented' joint replacement.

In some people with strong bones, it is possible to insert artificial joints without bone cement. This is called 'uncemented' or 'cementless' technique. This is commonly performed in the hip joints; not very popular in knees.

17. There are non-absorbable sutures, absorbable stiches, staplers and glues for closing the wound. Which one is better?

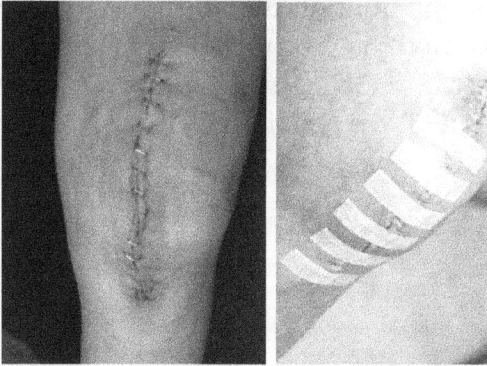

Figure 148

The kind of stitches used makes no real difference for the wound to heal unless it is misapplied. The stitch to be used on your knee depends entirely on the preference of your surgeon. Non-absorbable sutures and staplers are stronger but must be removed after two weeks. Absorbable stitches and glues are comparatively weaker but require no removal later. None of them makes any difference in the final results of your knee or hip replacement.

18. Which anesthesia is better?

Modern anaesthesia is safe and is administered in millions of people every year. Your anesthesiologist will examine and decide the best form of anaesthesia, depending on your body and medical conditions.

General and spinal anaesthesia are the two primary forms. Both of them administered successfully, commonly, and in large numbers. The anesthesiologist must assess you then and decide on the right type of anaesthesia for you. That said, you can have a successful joint replacement with any kind of anaesthesia.

19. How long does a surgery last?

The duration of the surgery always depends on the complexity of the procedure. On average, hip and knee replacements last for about 60 to 90 min. Mobilization, positioning, anaesthesia procedures, and pain-relieving procedures like nerve block will require a fair amount of additional time.

20. Will I have pain during surgery?

You will feel absolutely no pain during the whole procedure. The surgery cannot be performed if the pain is felt.

21. How many people are involved in my surgery?

These are the people involved in your surgery:

- A surgeon and one or two assistants
- An anaesthetist, his assistant, an anaesthesia technician

• A trained joint replacement nurse and a circulating-nurse, who will help everybody whenever needed. This number may vary from place to place.

22. Do I require blood transfusion?

Given the several advanced surgical techniques, not a lot of patients require blood transfusion lately. However, complex surgeries might still need a blood transfusion.

Blood transfusion can be done during surgery, but it is more commonly done post-surgery. If it is a case where both knees are replaced, then a blood transfusion is more commonly required.

23. What is a mini incision or a minimally invasive surgery?

Mini incision surgeries were developed to reduce the length of the scar and tissue damage due to operation. In hip and knee replacements, there have been no proven benefits of these techniques.

In fact, there may be complications purely because of these attempts. Therefore, these techniques remained unpopular and remained only as marketing tools to attract patients in many instances.

24. Is it laser or laparoscopic surgery?

Joint replacement surgeries are not laser or laparoscopic surgeries because joint replacement components are large and must be placed in the knee. This is possible only with larger cuts!

25. What is done to reduce pain?

Pain is controlled with several methods and their combinations called 'multimodal analgesia'. Common methods are a nerve block, epidural anaesthesia, local infiltrations, injections and pumps, and oral medications;

splinting and ice packs also reduce pain.

26. What is a nerve block?

A small catheter is placed directly on a nerve supplying sensation to the joint. This is done using an ultrasound scanner to localize the nerve. A small amount of local anaesthesia is delivered to the nerve directly using a pump. This can be used for two to three days.

27. How do you get exact size of my knee or hip replacement?

Implants are manufactured in different sizes which will be suitable for all sizes of people. Also, implants of all sizes will be available in the operation theatre every time a joint replacement surgery is undertaken.

28. What is computer aided navigation?

Computer-aided navigation helps the surgeon in preparing and positioning the implants accurately. Several studies have shown that component positioning is superior to conventional methods.

However, there is no statistical superiority in terms of function, pain relief, complications, or survival.

29. What is a robot-assisted joint replacement?

This is one of the latest advances in joint replacement surgery. A robotic arm is used to prepare the bone, using navigation principles. Robotic arm helps the surgeon to resect the bone more accurately and prevents the surgeon from inadvertently damaging the bone and tissues.

Early studies are encouraging, but long-term studies are still not available to confirm their superiority. Robot-assisted joint replacement has been discussed in detail in chapter 18.

30. Which is the best metal for knee or hip implants?

Commonly used materials are cobalt-chromium alloy, titanium, polyethylene, ceramic and oxinium. Metals and other materials can be used inside the human body only after robust clinical trials.

The most important factor to consider here is the duration of the use of these implants, and secondly, the number of people these implants have been successful in.

Most of the current generation implants are being used in millions of people for the last two decades. Cobalt-chromium for the knee is the most commonly used alloy and is also considered the safest.

31. Which is the best company for knee and hip implants?

There are several companies which make equally good implants, and no one can really be considered superior to the other. Companies such as Stryker, Johnson-Johnson, Zimmer, Smith & Nephew are commonly used all over the globe with comparable results.

32. What type of prosthesis /implant is used for my hip and how long will it last?

A variety of implants are used in knees and hips as described earlier—most of the implants on an average last about 20 years in over 90% of the people. Contrary to the common belief and commercial publications, there is not much of a difference between the companies and the type of implants.

After Surgery

33. What can I expect after knee replacement surgery?

After the knee replacement surgery, one should be able to go to the washroom all by themselves within three to four days of surgery, with or without the help of a cane. You will also be able to start all normal activities by six weeks.

That said, the total knees keep improving in terms of pain, flexibility and strength for a long time; it can take even up to 12 months. Post that, you should technically be able to lead a painkiller-free life and perform all daily activities with no concern whatsoever for many years.

34. How soon can I return to normal activities after surgery?

You can get back to normal activities in about six weeks after surgery. You can start all non-sport, non-impact activities such as driving, walking, swimming, and cycling by eight to 12 weeks.

35. My knee is warm postoperatively. Is this normal?

Yes, this is quite normal for about six to eight weeks. If it is excessively warm and remains warm for a longer time, the doctor can rule out the infection.

36. After surgery, is it normal for my knee to look larger than my other knee which has not had knee replacement surgery?

Replaced knees can look larger initially due to swelling. But everything should get back to normal in two to three months.

37. Is it normal to have numbness along the outer or lateral aspect of the incision?

Mild numbness on the outer side of the scar is very common. In some cases, people also develop small itchy skin rashes. This arises because small, hair-like, not very important sensory nerves have to be cut to reach your joint during surgery. They recover in about three to six months without any treatment.

38. After total knee or hip arthroplasty, what activities can I return to?

You can get back to all normal activities necessary for your age group. You are advised to refrain from heavy manual activities and sports. Cross leg sitting on the floor is generally avoided.

39. I have occasional clicking or clunking in my knee after surgery. Is this normal?

The clunking sounds are common; however, most of them aren't very significant. They occur when different surfaces of the artificial joint rub against each other. Earlier versions of the ceramic hip replacements usually cause these squeaking sounds. Most of them may annoy you but are medically safe and require no treatment if you have no pain.

40. How long should a patient remain in hospital after a knee or hip replacement?

If you are generally healthy, you can return home within three to four days after the surgery.

41. How soon can the patient stand up after a knee/hip replacement?

While some patients can stand up the same day of their

surgery, many others achieve this the next day. This also depends on the patient's age, medical conditions and their recovery from the anaesthesia.

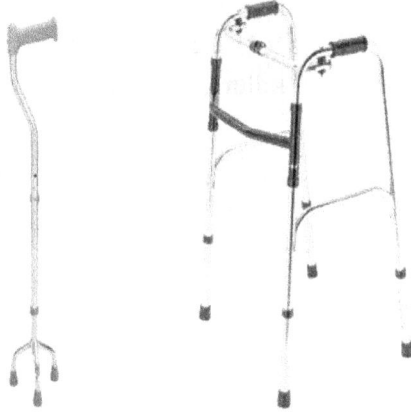

Figure 149: Walking aids

Suppose the patient is administered epidural or local block anaesthesia, then it may make their legs weaker, and the patient might not be able to walk properly until the effect of the anaesthesia is wholly waned off.

42. For how long will I have to use a walker?

After the hip and knee replacement surgery, walkers are used for about four to five days. Post that, a single stick will be adequate. However, patients who had both their joints replaced simultaneously (bilateral) may need a walker for about four weeks. Again, this duration also depends on the patient's age and strength. For example, someone who is 90 years old may need a walker permanently.

43. How soon can the patient be pain-free, after knee arthroplasty?

The patient will experience significant pain for about

four to six weeks post-surgery. The intensity of pain reduces with time, and he or she will start seeing significant changes in just two weeks.

However, if in rare cases, there exists a mild pain, simple measures like ice packs will work just fine. It would be best to avoid pain killers, given their side effects.

44. When can the patient go back to work?

The patients who undergo knee replacements are mostly retired and elderly. However, if the patient is still in service, desk jobs can be resumed in six weeks.

The patients can return to all other jobs after three months of surgery.

45. Can I travel overseas after the operation?

Yes, you can. But, make sure all the precautionary measures are in place. In fact, four to six weeks post-surgery, you can travel by road, flight or even by rail to any of your desired destinations.

46. Can I drive a car after surgery?

Yes, you can drive a car after six weeks of surgery. You can also cycle and ride a bike!

47. Will I be able to climb stairs?

Yes. You can start climbing up the stairs after three to four days of surgery. The physiotherapist in the hospital will help you with these activities.

48. Will I be able to kneel on my knee?

This is one thing that many patients find challenging. If you really require kneeling down, you can try with a pillow placed on the floor, under your knees to make it comfortable.

49. Can I go back to jogging?
Yes, most of the patients, depending on their physical health and age, can resume slow jogging.

50. Can I play tennis after my knee replacement?
Yes, most of the patients, depending on their physical health and age, do resume light sports.

51. Will I need to take any special precautions for the wound?
After the knee replacement, you will go home with a waterproof dressing on the operated wound. You can take a shower directly on the dressing.

You don't have to change the dressing at home until you return to see your surgeon after about two weeks.

52. How long will I have the swelling?
It is a gradual process. It may take up to six to eight weeks before the swelling is completely better. No medicines are required to reduce swelling.

53. What type of medication will I be taking post operation? Will I be taking it for long?
You will be taking a blood thinner for about four to six weeks. You will also be given some pain-killers. These are the only essential medicines. However, you might require other supporting medicines like calcium, vitamins, antacids, etc.

54. When is the suture removal?
After two weeks.

55. Do I have to do regular dressing after my discharge?

No regular dressing will be required after discharge. Your dressing will be changed on the day of discharge.

56. Should I continue my old medications?
Yes, most of the medications can be continued as before. This operation being a mechanical procedure, will not change your disease status. For example, you will not need to change your diabetes or hypertension medicines after a joint replacement.

57. Will I be put on a lifetime medication?
No maintenance medication is required. In fact, most of the patient need no medicines after four weeks of surgery.

58. Is it possible for my body to reject the new joint like a kidney transplant?
There is no rejection phenomenon in these metal joints because they are biologically inactive and immunologically inert.

59. Will I be on Immunosuppressant medications?
As joint replacement is a 'metal' with no immunological consequences. You will not require immuno-suppression medicines.

60. When can I start bathing?
You can start bathing in about two to three days post-surgery. You will be given a waterproof dressing that will allow you to take a shower directly on the knee or hip. But it would be best to avoid using bath-tubs until four to six weeks.

61. Do I need a physiotherapist when I return home, if so, for how long?

Most of the surgeons employ physiotherapy for two to four weeks. If you can do all your exercises on your own, a physiotherapist may not be required.

62. What do I do if I get loose stools or constipation?

There is no need to worry about this. Any illness that occurs after the knee replacement will be treated normally like any other person. Visit your general practitioner and get it treated in a normal passion. There is no need to change any of the standard medical treatments after joint replacements.

63. What do I do when I feel a burning sensation or heart burn?

An antacid medication works just fine when you have a burning sensation. This is usually prescribed after you are discharged from the hospital.

64. How long should I continue the antibiotics?

Only two or three doses of antibiotics will be administered after the joint replacement surgery. There will be no routine antibiotics from the second day onwards. You will not be taking any antibiotics after you go back home. Unnecessary use of antibiotics is generally avoided.

65. Do I need to apply a cold pack or a hot pack on the knee?

Cold packs are advised to reduce pain and swelling. You can use a normal cold pack from your freezer. Apply with a cloth or a tissue paper on the dressing or scar directly. Use it intermittently until you are comfortable.

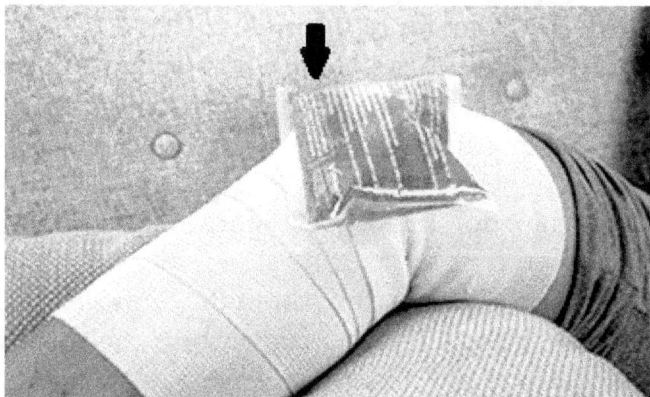

Figure 150: Ice packs on the knee

66. TED stockings, crepe bandage or elevation of limbs - Which is better?

You can practice all of them, as advised by your surgeons. They help reduce swelling and also prevent clotting complications in your operated leg. The only thing is, you have to continue practising these exercises for about four to six weeks or until you are fully mobile.

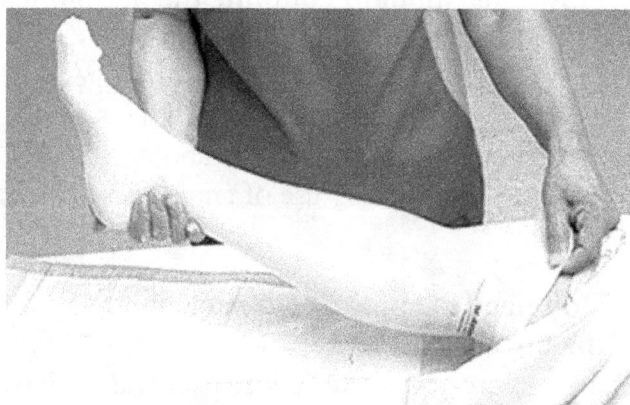

Figure 151: TEDS Stockings

67. What precautions should I take while flying and how early can I fly post-surgery?

Developing blood clots during long haul flights due to continuous sitting is one of the main fears of flying post-surgery.

Even though it is possible to travel after four weeks, it is best if you could avoid long-distance air travel for at least six to eight weeks.

While onboard, you should remember to exercise your ankles and take a walk inside the flight, every half hour. If you are at risk, you may be prescribed additional medications by your doctor.

68. When will I experience full benefit of my total knee or hip replacement?

You will experience full benefits around eight to twelve weeks after surgery. Both knees and hips continue to improve even after six to twelve months.

69. If I develop fever, what do I do?

If you have high body temperature, it might be because of a viral fever, sore throat, or urinary tract infection which are very common. However, a serious infection in your knee might also be the reason for high temperature.

Please note that if this fever continues for an unusual amount of time, especially with increasing pain, redness, and decreasing movements in the knee, you should consult your doctor immediately.

70. What can be done in case of breathlessness?

Breathlessness could be because of pulmonary embolism or the blood clots in your leg dispersed to your lungs. So, in such cases, you should visit the hospital immediately, as this is a serious condition calling for immediate treatment. Even though it could be from several other minor illnesses, you should contact your hospital immediately.

71. Do I continue my breathing exercises or spirometer exercises post-surgery? If so, for how long?

Breathing exercises will be taught to you when you are in the hospital if required. Patients can continue the same for about four to six weeks or even longer if needed.

72. How about my post-operative diet? Are there any specific diet plans that I should follow?

No, there will not be any diet restriction needed. On the day of the surgery, a simple liquid or a light diet is advised. You can gradually start with a regular diet. After going home, you should be able to eat everything you like unless you have diabetes or other medical conditions.

73. How do I manage my diabetes, hypertension or asthma after the surgery? Do I go back to my old medications?

Your other medical conditions will be monitored by a physician, as it is generally done in other patients. There will also be no routine changes in the medications even after you are sent home. However, immediately after surgery, you may have some variations in your blood sugar and hypertension due to the stress and pain involved.

74. Do I need to inform the doctor about the implant before I undergo any invasive procedure?

Yes. Doing so will help your doctor to give you an antibiotic if required.

75. What is the schedule for a review consultation?

You will have to visit the hospital on day 14 for the removal of stitches or staples. Further review is done after six weeks, followed by once after three months and finally, once every year. This protocol can change from hospital to hospital.

76. Am I allowed to consume alcohol or smoke after surgery?

Yes, there is no contraindication for sensible use of alcohol or smoking after joint replacement.

77. Should I have to take calcium and vitamin supplementation?

They may not have many roles to play in your recovery. However, you may receive them depending on the local hospital protocols or depending on your surgeon.

78. Will I be able to play high impact (skiing or golf or horse riding) sports?

They are possible if you are fit and young, but it is best to avoid high impact sports after joint replacements. Also, most of the patients who undergo joint replacement surgeries are elderly and need no such level of physical activities.

79. How many days should I stay in the hospital post- surgery?

You might have to stay in the hospital for three to four days. Some hospitals have started a rapid recovery program in some countries where patients are discharged on the same day or the very next day after surgery.

However, this is not routinely practised, and most elderly patients may not be the candidates to do that.

80. Postoperatively, will I require a blood transfusion? If yes, how do I acquire it?

A blood transfusion is rarely required. Your haemoglobin level in the blood will be checked by a simple blood test within 24 hours after the surgery and monitored later if needed. If haemoglobin is low (less than 7), you may need a blood transfusion. You will be able to procure the blood from the hospital blood bank.

81. How much can I walk at a stretch?

Once you are fully recovered from the surgery, there is no limit for your walking. People can resume a normal amount of walking, depending on their age.

However, you must remember that these surgeries are commonly performed in the elderly group of patients who may not be in the physical health required to take up extreme physical activities.

82. What is the best position for sleep after a knee replacement?

You can sleep in any position after a total knee replacement - supine, prone, or on either side. Sleep positions do not affect the recovery or the position of the knee prosthesis. However, it would be best if you do not overdo it.

83. What is the best position for sleep after a hip replacement?

A few precautions have to be taken after a hip replacement to prevent dislocations. Sleep on your back with your legs placed slightly wide apart; do not cross your legs. Keeping a pillow in between might make it easier and more comfortable (figure 152). You can also try sleeping on your sides; you can sleep on both sides.

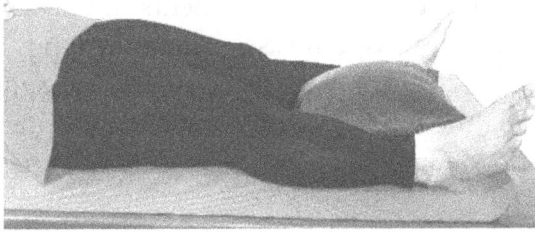

Figure 152

Sleeping on the operated side may take about six weeks or until the wound becomes painless. Sleeping on the operated side down is safer, and it will not affect your replaced joint. However, while sleeping sideways, especially with the non-operated leg down, keep a bulky pillow between the legs (figure 153). Sleeping on the stomach down is also allowed.

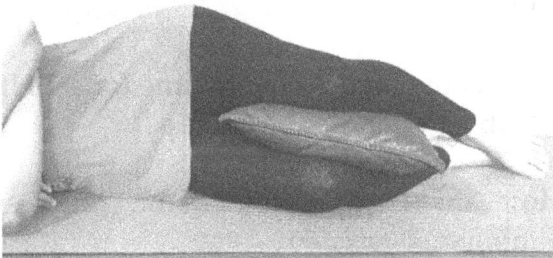

Figure 153

84. Will I able to use the regular commode, chairs and go on with my daily activities?

Yes, all this is possible once you have recovered from the operation, and this may take about six weeks. However, it is best to avoid using Indian style toilets even after six weeks.

85. Will there be complete movements at the hip joint after surgery?

Yes, normal ranges of movements are achievable in most people. However, in cases where the hip is severely affected, muscles are weak, and there's a tight tissue surrounding the hip, restoring complete movements may not be a possibility.

86. When can I lie down on my operated side after hip replacement?

You may lie down on your operated side in six to eight weeks post-surgery.

87. How efficient is physiotherapy post a THR? How long will it be administered for?

Hip, being a very muscular part of the body, does not need much of physiotherapy. However, if physical therapy is administered for three to four weeks, it may help strengthen your muscles, help you walk, and also correct your posture and gait.

88. What is the total recovery time for a THR?

It takes about eight to twelve weeks.

89. How do I get back home after surgery (ambulance or car?)

Most of the people may be able to go home in a normal car, sitting upright on the seat. However, some people with other medical conditions and those with both knees replaced together may need an ambulance.

90. Are obese patients equally satisfied after a joint replacement as other patients?

Yes. Several obese patients also benefit immensely

from joint replacement surgery. However, it is important to note that they might have more complications and that the joint replacement might not last long.

If the severity of the pain limits one's ability to function normally, a joint replacement can be considered. But, one should make every effort to reduce weight.

That said, some patients may not be able to lose weight due to their inability to walk and exercise and might need bariatric surgery.

91. How soon following THR will I be able to walk independently?

You will be able to walk in three to six weeks after surgery.

92. How often do I need to do my exercises?

About two to three times a day.

93. Do artificial joints set off the metal detectors in the airport?

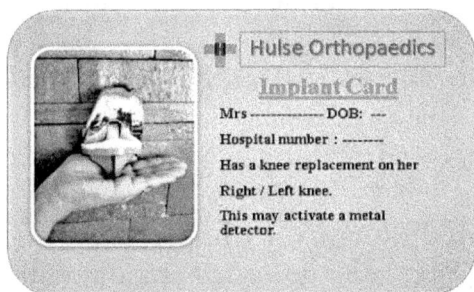

Figure 154: Implant card

Over 90% of implanted total hip and knee arthroplasty devices will set off an airport metal detector, and this may cause some delay and apprehension to some travellers. Hence a metal identification card or a letter can be issued by your surgeon.

94. Will I need a commode seat elevator?

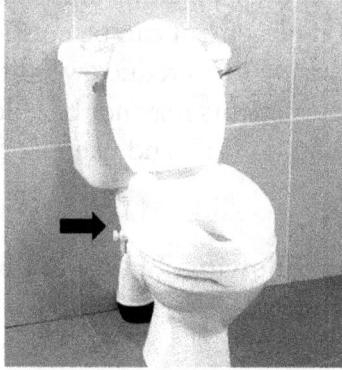

Figure 155: Toilet seat elevator

Toilet seat elevators are needed in the initial six weeks after hip or knee replacements, as sitting on a low chair could be difficult and uncomfortable.

95. Will I need a walking aid?

You will need a pair of crutches or a walking frame for the first week or two. Then a single walking stick should be adequate. Depending on the age and general health, you will be able to ambulate without support in four to six weeks.

96. Should I modify my house in any way?

No. There are no such modifications needed. However, a toilet seat elevator and an accessible washroom will be required, as mentioned earlier.

97. Does the healing process depend on the weather?

Weather makes absolutely no difference in the healing

process. Replacements are done throughout the year, in all weather conditions with equal success.

98. Should I switch to a ground floor room post-surgery?

This isn't generally needed as most people manage to take a few steps within a week or two.

99. Will I need help with household chores?

Not much help is really required. If anything, you might need some help in cooking, cleaning, and doing other chores for about four weeks.

100. Do I need a rehab or a nursing home?

Rehabs and nursing homes are not needed in everyone's case. Those patients who have no family support and require supervised medical care, or frail older adults needing longer rehabilitation may need a step-down facility like a nursing home or a care home.

Other patients can manage at their own homes within their existing social and family support.

101. How much can I bend my knee post-surgery?

The total knee can bend about 110 degrees on average. Usually, a minimum of 95 degrees of bending is required for daily activities like climbing stairs, getting up from a chair and walking on uneven surfaces. This is the reason why people after knee replacements have no restrictions on their daily activities.

102. How long does a joint replacement last?

Most of the joint replacements (hip and knee) last for about 20 years in over 90% of the patients.

INDEX

www.ingramcontent.com/pod-product-compliance
Lightning Source LLC
Chambersburg PA
CBHW050110280326
41933CB00010B/1035